SLEEPLESS CHILDREN:
A HANDBOOK FOR PARENTS

SLEEPLESS CHILDREN: A HANDBOOK FOR PARENTS

BY DR. DAVID HASLAM

LONG SHADOW BOOKS
PUBLISHED BY POCKET BOOKS NEW YORK

A Long Shadow Book published by
POCKET BOOKS, a division of Simon & Schuster, Inc.
1230 Avenue of the Americas, New York, N.Y. 10020

ISBN: 0-671-54302-4

First Long Shadow Books printing January, 1985

Originally published in Great Britain by
Judy Piatkus (Publishers) Limited, London

10 9 8 7 6 5 4 3 2 1

For
Barbara, Katy and Christopher

ACKNOWLEDGMENTS

◆

I could not have written this book without the assistance and advice of a great many people. In particular I would like to thank all those parents of sleepless children who have written or talked to me about their experiences, all the authors whose research I have quoted, and the many representatives of official organizations who have taken time to let me know their views. I am also most grateful to Anne Palmer for typing the manuscript, and last, but not least, to my family for their encouragement and tolerance during the time I was writing it.

CONTENTS

◆

PART IV

HOW TO SURVIVE

SLEEPLESS CHILDREN: A HANDBOOK FOR PARENTS

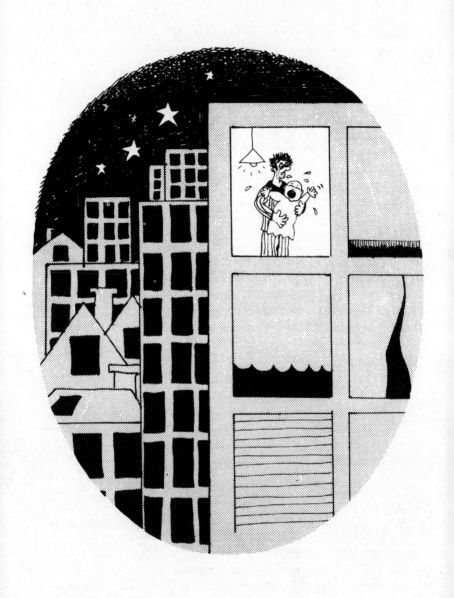

Introduction

◆

There is something very lonely about 3 A.M. Sitting in a young child's bedroom while he screams at the top of his voice, a parent can feel that no one else in the world can be suffering quite as much. The moon may be shining, and the stars twinkling, but for the parent of a sleepless child the hours of darkness become a waking nightmare. To make matters worse, when the parent, bleary-eyed and exhausted, tells friends about the problem the usual response is either disbelief or criticism. Disbelief because if she were telling the truth, how can she explain that her child is running around looking happy, healthy, and totally refreshed. Criticism because everyone—or at least everyone who has not suffered—knows that if you were only to bring children up "correctly" then the problem would never occur. It is enough to drive parents to despair.

Of course, there really are no such beings as "sleepless children". All children get some sleep, and nearly all get enough sleep. What matters is the effect on the parents, and if you have been woken night after night, month after month, then it can certainly feel like your child is sleepless. I make no apology for appearing to exaggerate in the title of this book. Anyone who has suffered will know exactly what it means, and this is one of those rare areas of life where it is remarkably difficult for someone who

13

has not suffered to truly understand the intensity of the emotions that can be stirred up.

Unfortunately, a majority of the books and articles that have been written on the subject come across as distinctly unsympathetic and unhelpful. The fact that most of their authors had never spent an exhausting night with a wakeful toddler stands out a mile, if only because much of the advice they offer is remarkable in its uselessness. Many parents reading such books or articles end up feeling even more inept and guilty than before. The rare exceptions are those writers who have suffered themselves, and they stand out like beacons in the dark.

I claim to be no great expert on the scientific intricacies of sleep disorders. In fact my chief qualifications to write on the subject are Katy and Christopher, my children. They nearly drove my wife, Barbara, and me to despair when we heard yet again their plaintive cries at three in the morning. The more I read about the subject, the more aware I became of its complexities, and the more parents I met whose stories matched our own. Studies have shown that 20% of parents of young children have these problems, and I realized that tens of thousands of parents were awake night after night, and that our story was far from being the horrific exception that I had once thought.

When I began to research this book I became very aware that many parents were reassured to know that their doctor had suffered in a similar way. Indeed, I received a large number of lengthy letters from parents of sleepless children, many of whom described their encounters with various health care and social work professionals. Over and over again they wrote that they received the most understanding and sympathy from professionals who had suffered themselves. One woman told how she had poured all her problems out to her doctor, only to have him pour all his own children's sleeping problems out to her. She left, realizing that compared to his sleepless night she had not lived. The medical professions would normally frown on such a consultation. When it comes to physical or psychiatric problems they would be right, but with a problem as common as this, the realization that you are not alone and that even your doctor may not have the answer can be remarkably reassuring. As another mother told me, "As I left his office, my doctor called out that if ever I found out how to make my children sleep, would I go back and tell him so that he could sort his own out. I found his honesty tremendously refreshing, and I respected him for it."

The danger for doctors who have suffered themselves is that they will assume everyone else's problems are the same as theirs. This is not the case. There are very many causes of sleeplessness, types of sleeplessness, and solutions to the problem. Each one needs considering individually, even though the frustrations and emotions that result may be very similar. It is also essential that health care professionals find out what parents mean by sleeplessness. For example, a mother might leap out of bed every time she hears her child whimper, rush noisily to his room and put the light on, only to wake him up. Such a parent is creating a problem for herself, and needs quite different guidance from that given to the parent whose child spontaneously wakes up crying every night. Unfortunately many people in the past have been aware of the first, overanxious, group and have assumed that all the other parents were the same. It is not surprising therefore that they have little sympathy for the great mass of sleepless parents.

I had never even considered the problem before Katy was born, seven years ago. It was never mentioned at medical school, and not surprisingly I had never come across it during my time working in hospitals. Like all medical students I had studied child development and had read rather fuzzy descriptions of how the average newborn baby sleeps nearly all the time between feedings. Who was I to disbelieve the experts?

Katy soon changed all that. Even as a tiny baby she hardly ever slept in the day. She would lie in a small hammock-style chair and watch my wife. At that age she could not focus accurately on what Barbara was doing, nor understand a word that was said to her, but as long as she was nearby she was happy. I remember arriving home early when she was only a couple of months old to find Barbara talking to her about how she was baking a cake. She was perfectly happy, but never wanted a daytime nap. Two lessons became rapidly apparent. First, in the case of at least one child who appeared otherwise perfectly normal, the books were wrong. Second, and more interesting, was the fact that no one who did not visit us actually believed us.

When it came to bedtime the books were wrong too. Katy woke every single night until she was two years old, with only one glorious exception. When she wouldn't settle at bedtime and screamed, it became pointless to leave her there as the books suggested. A healthy child can scream for an incredibly long time. We were living in a small apartment and to follow such advice, even if it had worked, would have been antisocial in the extreme. Instead, we would sit by her crib reading until she eventually dropped off. When this failed, we found a ride in the car usually got her to sleep—until we switched the engine off. The only reason I don't feel embarrassed admitting such nighttime adventures is that I have met so many other parents who have done the same, doctors included.

On occasions when she woke in the night and we were both exhausted we would take her into our bed. She usually slept wonderfully, but her wriggling kept my wife awake and so was a less than perfect answer. In fact, the solitary occasion when she slept right through the night without waking was when we spent a night camping when she was seven months old. It was bitterly cold, but she wore warm pajamas and did not move all night. It was so unusual that Barbara and I lay awake wondering what was wrong. Had she died? Was she still breathing? Whatever had happened?

Eventually she woke happy and bright at 8 o'clock. For a long time I assumed it was the clean country air, or the novelty of camping. Now I am less sure. Could it have been the closeness to her parents that our tiny tent made inevitable?

We also discovered another curious fact that medical school had never taught me, and science has yet to explain. In the late afternoon she would clearly be getting tired, and yet five minutes curled up on a chair sucking her thumb would totally restore her energy for several hours. It does not make sense, but it happened.

Shortly before her second birthday things gradually began to improve. She didn't go to sleep readily, but was happy to sit and look at picture books by herself, and her night waking gradually faded out. My wife was then pregnant. Everyone, including ourselves, said it could not happen twice. Katy might not have slept much, but the new baby would.

A week after Katy's first complete run of seven undisturbed nights, Christopher was born. He was even worse. He was the most miserable, tearful, whining, crying baby imaginable. Every night he woke two or three times. Every day Barbara despaired of ever finding a way to calm him down. He hated his baby carriage and screamed in the car. At night Barbara would tell me as we lay there listening to him, "You'd better go again, I think I'll kill him." Almost every parent I have spoken to on this subject has felt exactly the same. Life can become an utter misery.

Again, we occasionally found that he would sleep reasonably well in our bed, but if Katy found out in the morning she would inevitably wake the next night and come in for a cuddle herself. We just could not win. We didn't mind them being there, but with four in a bed someone had to give. Usually the morning found Barbara or myself asleep in Katy's bed.

Daytimes improved dramatically when Chris was seven months old and began to walk. He became cheerful and, at last, fun to know. At that time we again went camping and I found the only advantage of having a sleepless child that I know. Chris would wake at 5:30 A.M. and sing. We were in a crowded campsite and such activity is hardly encouraged. So he and I would get dressed and I would take him for a walk in the country. On other days we would go and watch the fishing boats come in, and would then sit in a fisherman's cafe as I drank a large cup of coffee and watched the locals gather. They must have thought I was crazy. Who in their right mind takes a seven-month-old baby out for a walk at that hour? The parent of a sleepless child, that's who.

As Kate and Christopher got older things slowly improved. Nursery school helped tire them out, and eventually the problem disappeared. Often they lie awake for hours reading or singing, but if they are happy we do not mind. Christopher is now just five, and last week we had the first occasion when he went to the bathroom in the night and did not consider it necessary to call into our room on the way back to tell us he'd finished. We were very grateful, even though we had heard him anyway.

During the time that our two children were not sleeping I began to hear of more and more parents who had the same problem but felt isolated and exhausted. It slowly began to dawn on me just how large the problem is, an impression confirmed by reading the several excellent research reports that have looked at such childhood problems, many of which I quote at length in this book.

It was at this stage that I wrote a short magazine article on the problem, and in the weeks that followed received a huge number of deeply moving letters from exasperated parents. "I don't believe it," wrote one. "I didn't believe anyone was ever going to take sleepless nights seriously." The letters, each one often running to over ten pages in length, made me realize the tip of the iceberg that my personal experiences represented. I have quoted these letters extensively throughout the book, and am most grateful to their authors. Almost every letter finished with the comment that the writer felt relieved at having got the matter off his or her chest, and I hope such relief was longlasting. They, too, will now realize that they are not alone.

Throughout the book I have called the child "he." The only reason for this is that it is far less longwinded than writing "he or she" every time. The same reason applies when talking about the parents. Because more mothers wrote to me, and more mothers than fathers get up at night, I opted to say "mother" instead of "mother and father." This does not mean that I am implying that child rearing is solely the mother's job. Children are for sharing, and sharing the pleasure means sharing the problems.

In practice this meant that in our family when Christopher woke in the night both Barbara and I would desperately pretend to be asleep, all the while realizing that the other was doing just the same. Eventually one of us would give in, and the other would roll over, pretending to have woken at precisely that moment, and offer to go. By then it was too late! It's easy to pretend to be chivalrous when you know your partner has already got up! It is therefore with that thought that I dedicate this book to all those parents who know the frustration of repeatedly getting up on a cold dark night to a sleepless child. I know how you feel.

What I will be doing in this book is considering the various types of sleep disturbance, illustrating them with the experiences of sufferers, and explaining as much as possible about why they occur. I will offer my suggestions for helping you to cope. Some you will have tried, some will sound obvious, and others obscure. Nevertheless, I will mention as many different factors as possible in the hope that they throw light on an aspect of your own problem that you have overlooked. There will also be various suggestions and theories that you will not have heard of and may wish to try. Indeed, you may find that there is some part of your management of your child that is actually creating the problem, or you may find—as frequently happens—that the child is sleeping badly despite your doing everything right.

By the end of the book you will have considered almost every angle of the problem of sleepless children, and with luck will have found your answer. Whatever else happens you will at least realize that you are far from alone. There are an awful lot of us who know just how you feel.

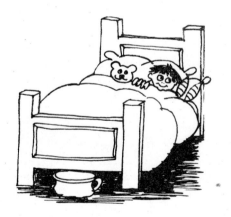

SLEEP
AND
SLEEPLESSNESS

♦ **1** ♦

Sleepless Children—
Who Suffers?

"It never seems to end. You wouldn't believe what that does to you. Every night you go to bed knowing that there is no way that you'll go through the night without being disturbed. You lie there waiting for him to cry. Your sleep is fitful. Even when he does sleep solidly for a few hours, you're so tied up with the sheer frustration of it all that you can't relax. It made me want to scream."

Mother of a two-year-old

It is a pity that babies don't read books. It is even more of a pity that they can't tell the time. If only they could learn all the latest theories about sleep requirements before being dispatched to their families, then the problem of sleeplessness wouldn't occur. Unfortunately, they arrive totally ignorant of what they are expected to do, and naively unaware that it is the family that has to adjust to them, and not them to the family.

Indeed, if only the effect on the family could be ignored then it is generally agreed by most experts that babies and children almost always get enough sleep.[1,2] Doctors are rarely worried about how much sleep a child gets, but are more concerned with how much sleep its parents are getting. If your child wakes up twenty times in the night but doesn't cry or wake you, and is otherwise happy and healthy, then there is no problem. However,

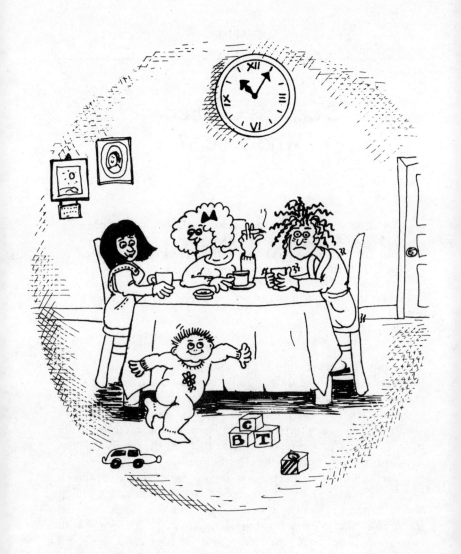

if he wakes only once every night, but will not settle without you getting up to him, then you may indeed feel that you have very real difficulties. This book is directed at all parents who are unhappy about their child's sleeping habits. You may find as you read on that you do not really have anything to be concerned about. If so, the problem as such may cease to exist, even though your child's sleep has stayed exactly the same. I will not be attempting to define any more precisely what a "sleepless child" is. If you feel you have got one, then read on.

Children vary tremendously in the amount of sleep that they seem to need. For instance, it has been estimated that around a quarter of all pre-school children persist in waking at night (see Chapter 3). Nevertheless, it is extremely rare to come across an adult who has suffered because he or she did not get enough sleep as a child. Some children sleep happily right through the night, with additional naps of an hour or so during the day, while others only sleep solidly at night for a couple of hours at a time, and rarely seem to need a daytime nap. Despite the differences, both types of children will grow up equally healthy, happy and bright. If children could be left to their own devices and did not need the attention of adults, then no one would really be the least concerned about whether they sleep or not.

When problems do arise, they almost always stem from the fact that the parents of a sleepless child need their sleep at a time that doesn't suit the child. The child does not realize that it is antisocial to wake at three in the morning and want to play. If the parent could adapt his or her life to be awake when the child is awake, and asleep when he is asleep, then the child's waking would not cause any problems. Because adults live by a clock that is, initially at least, meaningless to the child, stresses arise. For example, the mother quoted at the start of this chapter had always gone to bed at 11 P.M. before her child was born. She would read for fifteen minutes, then sleep peacefully till 7:30 in the morning. This was her pattern and she liked it. Sleeping like this she felt bright and energetic, able to face the world with confidence.

When Michael, her first baby, arrived, this pattern was completely disrupted. He would go to sleep reluctantly at seven, wake at eleven, and play or want feeding or cuddling till midnight. When he eventually dropped off and his mother managed to get to bed—tired and resentful—her sleep would be disturbed again at about 2:30, and she would eventually be woken in the morning at six. Michael would be fine. She would be shattered. Tired and frustrated, she spent the day wondering where she had gone so terribly wrong.

Michael showed most of the different types of sleep disturbance that I will be examining in detail in later chapters. The major difficulties that parents have to deal with start with a reluctance to go to bed, and difficulties in going to sleep. Equally exhausting is the child who wakes repeatedly during the night, or whose sleep is disturbed in other ways such as sleep-walking or nightmares. Finally, there are the children who wake far earlier than their parents would wish. Each of these patterns poses its own problems, and disrupts family life in its own special way.

Sleep difficulties are by no means confined to young babies. In a magnificently thorough piece of research, John and Elizabeth Newson interviewed the parents of over 700 one-year-olds.[3] They found that 35% of mothers had reported that they had been woken at some time during the night preceding the interview, and in almost all the cases it had been necessary for one of the parents to get up to see the child. Thirty-five percent. That's an awful lot of tired parents. Even more interesting is the fact that 16% of the babies were reported to be waking regularly every night.

The Newson findings are not isolated ones. Almost every survey of child behavior has pinpointed sleeping problems as being of immense concern to parents. A study by psychologists in 1973 found that regular night-waking was the biggest problem faced by the parents of fourteen-month-olds.[4] As a family physician I have certainly been impressed by how frequently parents mention their disturbed nights, and a detailed study in 1972 found that four out of ten children between the ages of six months and five years had some sort of sleep problem.[5] Thankfully after the age of five the problem usually begins to lessen, though not in every case. Many children over this age do still wake but are old enough to get out a book or play with toys. With luck they will have developed enough social sensitivity to leave their parents asleep and unaware.

There is no doubt whatsoever that sleep problems are remarkably common. It is therefore extraordinary how isolated and alone most suffering parents feel. When I began to research this subject I received a huge number of letters from parents. A typical opening paragraph read, "I was so pleased to read that I am not the only person in the world with two terrors who wake me up numerous times in the night." Another wrote, "The worst thing I found is thinking we were the only ones." And another, "I read of your research with immense relief. I didn't think anyone else had these problems."

One particularly moving letter told of the sheer frustration of night after night of disturbed sleep and the conviction that the writer's friends couldn't possibly have the same difficulties. What summed up for me the impact that this experience had on her was her opening paragraph. "Hearing of your research brought back memories, hardly dimmed by the passage of 15 years, of so many disturbed nights, that I felt moved to write." This is no trivial experience. Sleepless children cannot be thought of as just a passing nuisance; even though, thankfully, the problem itself always passes eventually. The memories may not.

The effects of repeatedly disturbed nights on parents can be immense. One mother told me, "The trouble is, it snowballs. The first few weeks are tolerable. You've got a new baby. You expect a bit of trouble. You're still optimistic and all your friends say, 'Don't worry, he'll soon settle down.' The weeks go by and he doesn't settle down. You get tired and resentful. You're too tired for a sex life, and anyway, bedtime is too precious to waste on sex. You just want to sleep. You start to get crabby with the baby and your husband. My husband slept through it all and couldn't see the problem. He told me to see the doctor about the sex business, but it was just the sleep. All I needed was a decent sleep."

This frustration can frequently become an overwhelming part of one's life. It's bad enough not getting the sleep. To have friends whose children seem to be little angels, who sleep peaceful, undisturbed sleep from six in the evening to seven in the morning, can seem like sheer punishment. As this same mother said to me, "What makes it even worse is that whenever you complain about the little monster not sleeping, he will run about as bright as a button and make you feel like an absolute liar. You can see your friends thinking, 'What a lot of fuss. No child that happy lies awake screaming all night.' Even when I went to the doctor he said that the child looked fine and there was nothing to worry about. Couldn't he see the bags under my eyes? I could have wept."

The child himself may not appear to an outsider to pose a particularly great problem. He may only wake for a very short while, but this may be enough to cause the parents immense distress. I remember a father telling me, "It's not that Jenny would lie awake for hours. She's not too bad that way. Once we get up and go to her she's asleep again within minutes. The trouble is that we are not. Once we're awake, neither my wife nor I can get back to sleep easily. When we do, it's often only for an hour or so before Jenny has another of her waking spells and we're up again. It's maddening." In Part Four of the book I will look at the various ways in which parents like these can best survive their ordeal.

It is not only the parents who suffer. Other children in the family can be disturbed and frustrated by the noise in the early hours. It is bad enough if it is a noise down the corridor. When the noise shares your bedroom it is no fun at all. Brothers and sisters will inevitably suffer from the heightened tension in the family that results from exhausted parents. They can find themselves shouted at for trivial misdemeanors solely because their parents' patience has finally worn out. They are rarely old enough to understand what is going on. They just wonder why a minor offense like spilling some milk at breakfast gets them screamed at. It cannot seem at all fair. Small wonder that new babies are not always welcomed unreservedly by older brothers and sisters.

Neighbors, too, may feel the same way. If you live in the depths of the countryside in a thick-walled isolated house, then you are spared this aspect of sleepless children, but a majority of young families these days live in small thin-walled houses or apartments. The embarrassment at imagining the neighborhood listening to one's "failure" can be almost overwhelming. As Carol, the mother of a very restless nine-month-old, told me, "You think everybody must be listening. Whenever Simon wakes I feel sure that the whole neighborhood can hear him. I can't stand the thought of waking everyone else up. I'm sure they must lie there cursing me every night. If we were miles from anywhere I don't think his crying would bother me half as much. It just sounds so deafening in the early hours."

Daytime sleep, or the lack of it, can also cause problems. The amount of sleep that children need in the daytime varies considerably. While this book deals mainly with bedtime problems, there is no doubt that parents of children who hardly ever sleep in the day may also have considerable difficulties. So do those whose children don't stick to a set routine in the day. Adults tend to live their lives by the clock. The pattern is set. Lunch is at one. Supper at seven. Children are picked up from school at 3:30. The young child has no concept of this. Instead of behaving considerately by having a nap while Mom prepares lunch, he insists on being played with as she tries to peel the potatoes with her one available hand—no easy task. When she has to go out, he drops off to sleep in his crib. Other children suffer too. The demanding wakeful baby will effectively stop his mother from playing with brothers and sisters, causing guilt on one side and jealously on the other. More frustrations. More questions.

All in all, the catalog of problems is now very familiar. The child doesn't sleep at convenient times. The parents get tired. The tiredness turns to tension, guilt, and frustration. Sex lives all but disappear. Indeed, a huge proportion of the letters I received mentioned the effect of sleepless nights on the sex life of the writer. One mother wrote splendidly about this. "Apart from the raging anger and hostility which a parent has to cope with if his or her sleep is constantly interrupted—I used to liken it to a kind of brainwashing technique—there is the problem of sex which adds its quota of tension to an already rumbling volcano! Naturally, it is very hard to have free, open, joyous, harmonious, adventurous sexual relations if they are interrupted invariably by the patter of tiny feet. It is a very sticky problem. If only parents could be provided with at least four free weekends away from home every year then marital harmony would improve beyond all expectations."

There is certainly no doubt that a sleepless child is one of the world's most effective contraceptives. This puts tremendous stress on the marriage, and I know of several families where the exhaustion and frustration of repeated sleepless nights was a major factor in the breakup of the marriage. Of course, the child inevitably reacts to the increased tension in the family by sleeping even less well. Of all the vicious circles, this is one of the most vicious.

It is no wonder that poor sleep in children is often one of the last straws before a parent batters a child. Few parents can condone such action. Even fewer have not looked at their screaming child after he has seemed to settle for the fifth time at three in the morning, only to wake as you tiptoe to the door, without wanting to fling him out of the window and at last get some peace. Every parent understands such feelings, and the huge majority of parents never harm their children. Nevertheless, feeling can run very high. Sally, mother of three sleepless preschoolers, wrote of her feelings toward the eldest: "Not only did I have to cope with sleepless nights, but I also had to cope with my feelings of hatred for my little girl. I had to do something. I took her to the hospital on at least six occasions pretending there was something wrong or that she'd had a fit. The truth is that I saw my beautiful daughter as an ugly nasty monster who was ruining a lot of lives, and I hated her nearly as much as I loved her."

Parents who actually cause nonaccidental injuries to their children often have other very serious problems and lack the safety valves that other parents use. But even so, poor sleep can be a very major factor. Parents who abuse their children often have very high and unrealistic expectations of his behavior and development, believing him to be more abnormal than he actually is.[6] Such parents are usually very demanding and rigid, and with such families the fuse seems almost inevitably primed for explosion when a child fails to sleep. Those whose fuses are a little longer can still know how they feel.

A child abuse consultant told me that he found, particularly with middle-class parents, that sleepless nights are continually referred to, as is the frustration felt when professional advisers belittle the problem.

In a professional guide to helping families where nonaccidental injury is a problem there appears the comment, "There comes that dreadful moment in every parent's life when love and a desire to care for the child is mixed with incredible disappointment, anger, and even hate."[7] It is surprising not that there are so many battered children, but that there are so few.

Happy families need parents who get their sleep. One mother made her feelings very clear. "By the time Thomas was a year old we were obsessed with the idea of sleep. Even our own families found us unbearably dull as we could talk or think of little else. We decided that if this was parenting, you could keep it! My husband had a vasectomy before Thomas was two."

That last sentence says so much. It seems tragic that such a problem can cause such immensely powerful emotions. If only more people could understand how common their experiences are, and how normal their emotional reactions of disappointment and failure can be, then parenthood might be viewed in a far more realistic and honest light. As it is, society's attitudes to child rearing are sometimes extraordinary. It has always struck me as rather odd that in our society we call a baby who doesn't cause any problems a "good baby." If he sleeps all night, never throws his food, never hits the cat, never sticks his fingers in the electric sockets, and never spills his milk all over you, then he is a perfect child. Perhaps the ultimate in "good" babies, going by all the usual definitions, would be the one who was almost permanently unconscious. The fact that a child may be anything but "good," and yet is developing entirely normally, seems to count for little in the morning coffee chatter of mothers. The rather slow, uninspiring, quiet, and apathetic baby is looked at as "ever so good," and "not a bit of trouble." The inquisitive, moody, mischievous, bright child causes far more problems. I always feel very sad when I hear mothers answer the question "Is he a good baby?" with "Yes, he's wonderful. I hardly know he's there."

There is another unfortunate consequence of this attitude. Once society has said that a child who sleeps all night is "good," then it is hardly surprising that many parents reach the apparently logical conclusion that if their child does not sleep, either he must be a "bad" child or they are "bad" parents. They end up not only feeling tired and exhausted, but guilty and incompetent as well. As we will see over and over again in this book, parents regularly ignore the advice of the established experts. Indeed, they frequently say when describing how they try to cope with a problem, "Of course, I know it's wrong, but . . . " However eminent the authority, if advice sounds wrong and does not seem to be either common sense or humane, then it must surely be poor advice. Parents are very often given unrealistic expectations about sleeping times and ineffective advice in managing the problem, and then they wonder why they feel tired and confused.

One mother wrote to me quoting a number of books she had read on child care problems, and she said of the advice she had read, "I now feel quite certain it is nonsense, though I must admit that I and several friends took it all quite seriously at one point. Guilt seemed to plague me and my conscientious friends and often deterred us from asking for the help we needed."

There are no easy universal answers to sleep problems. No one can guarantee that any single method will work with your child. Every child, and every parent, is different. Some of the advice that I offer may not suit the way you want to bring up your child. If so, and if you understand the reasons behind your decision and my suggestion, then do not feel you are wrong. You know your child.

• 2 •

Normal Sleep

Sleepless nights, as we have seen, can cause parents tremendous problems. Any consideration of sleep disturbance must look at "normal" sleep, and many parents want guidance on how long their child should sleep at any given age.

Many books and articles have been published with tables and charts that give definite guidelines as to what is "normal." These tables certainly have the virtue of simplicity. Many people appreciate being given definite hard-and-fast rules about child care. If you read, as it is stated in one popular handbook for parents, that "the average six-year-old should sleep for ten hours each night," then at least you have a clearly stated rule against which you can measure your own child. If your child seems to be following the rules then you will be perfectly happy.

Life is not that simple. What are you supposed to do if your child does not do what the book says? It is easy for experts to cause immense concern among parents who think that because their child does not measure up to the averages then there must be something wrong either with their child or with their parental management. This problem occurs in many areas of child development. It is therefore absolutely essential that you read any such statements with one golden rule in mind: Beware of Averages.

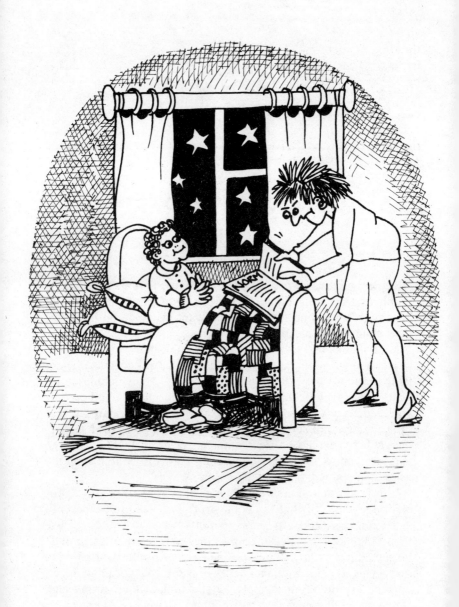

If, for example, you read that the average child walks three steps at thirteen months of age, then do remember that this means that 50% of children will be earlier than this, and 50% later. That is all it means. Unfortunately it also leads half the parents to believe their child is wonderfully gifted because he or she walked sooner, and half the parents to become extremely worried because their child is apparently "slow."

Do not, please, make this mistake. The sort of statistics that the sleep researchers have come up with are not a value judgement. They are a guide to how another group of children slept. Perhaps even more importantly, if your child is sleeping more or less than average, do remember that he hasn't read the research and isn't aware of his mistake.

In the example I quoted earlier, it was stated that "the average six year old should sleep for ten hours each night." The word "should" is completely out of place. It may be true that the "average" child does sleep that long, but this does not mean that harm will come to a child who does not.

Before looking in some detail at the discoveries that have been made about "normal" sleep in children, there is one other complicating factor to remember. One of the problems in researching this kind of topic is getting hold of subjects to examine. As a result more research tends to be performed on the newborn, who are captive in a hospital setting, and on children in institutions. As we will see later, such children tend to have a very different incidence of sleep problems than the child in a family home. It is not always possible to say that the results which such research has come up with are directly applicable to the average child in a normal family, but nevertheless some definite observations have been made that apply to almost all children.

In particular, a number of interesting discoveries have been made on how an infant's sleep pattern develops. Far from being haphazard, a newborn infant does have a very definite rhythm of eating, sleeping and waking. After birth the cycle almost fits the twenty-four hour cycle of the older child and adult—the circadian rhythm—but is often twenty-three or twenty-five hours, or occasionally even longer. Over the first three to four months the baby's regular rhythm gradually begins to fit the twenty-four hour cycle that the rest of us live by.

As far as parents are concerned, the ideal development in the sleep pattern is for most of the sleep to occur at night and most of the wakefulness during the day. In looking at this, it was found that the average new-born child sleeps for sixteen–seventeen hours, and the average sixteen-week-old child sleeps for fourteen–fifteen hours.[1] However, a significant change occurred in the length of individual sleeping spells. In the first week the average longest sleep is four hours. By sixteen weeks the average longest sleep is eight and a half hours. With any luck this long spell will coincide with the parents' sleeping time. If it does, then everyone is happy and you wouldn't be reading this book. If it doesn't— and it is a common occurrence that these averages do not show up—then you've got problems.

As well as considering the lengths of periods of sleep, it is also possible to consider how the so-called "average" child's sleep varies from age to age in terms of the number of sleeping periods. Most new-born babies sleep almost all the time, but by three months their day includes three or four sleeping periods. By the time they are a year old there are only two or three sleeps in the twenty-four hours, and by three years old very many children only sleep at night, though others need an afternoon nap till they are four or five years old.

It is useless to provide more rigid guidelines than these. These are averages, and some children will sleep more and others less. They throw some light on the normal development of sleeping habits, but are only an observation on what usually happens. If your child does not match this pattern he will almost certainly not come to harm, and for this reason I am very reluctant to lay down any more dogmatic rules on this aspect of sleep.

While researching this aspect of sleep I came across a number of well-respected child care guides that gave detailed descriptions of what the average child is thought to do at any given age with regards to settling down at night, waking up in the night, or napping in the day. However, if you read that the average three-year-old is happy to rest in his bed during the day without making a fuss and your child does not, what does the information prove? The parents' guide which gives that information also says that the four-year-old rarely takes things to bed with him and that the fifteen-month-old is put to bed easily. If such information is correct, what value is it?

Too many parents follow their children's progress against check lists that will either make them undeservedly proud or unnecessarily ashamed. Certain developmental landmarks are, of course, useful in assessing general development. But on the subject of sleeping problems they are of marginal interest at best.

The fact is that children vary in their sleeping patterns almost as much as adults. This is not just a casual observation. In 1976 an interesting report was published.[2] Analyzing individual differences in the time children spend asleep, the authors came to the conclusion, after an immense amount of technical study, that infants vary tremendously not only in how long they sleep but also in how restless they are, in how deeply they sleep, and in how much they move. They felt that one of the major factors leading to these differences was the infant's personality. In other words, different children sleep differently. This seems to be another example of science proving what every parent knows. But at least such a study sets out in black and white the fact that children may not fit with the child care guide averages and yet be perfectly normal.

In the next few chapters I will be considering some of the factors that affect a child's sleep, and the different forms that sleep problems can take. To explain many of these—in particular, nightmares, bed-wetting, sleepwalking, and similar difficulties—I will need to refer to some of the more technical aspects of our current knowledge about sleep. It is also important that parents understand something about their own sleep and how this can vary, and the effects of sleep deprivation.

Until recently surprisingly little was known about sleep, and modern sleep research dates from 1952. In April 1952, a young physiology graduate named Eugene Aserinsky, who is now thought of as one of the fathers of scientific sleep analysis, was researching at Chicago University using the EEG. The EEG, or electroencephalogram, is a recording of the electrical impulses of the brain, painlessly made by placing electrodes on the head. While performing a series of these measurements, Aserinsky made an observation which countless sleepless men and women must have made while looking at their sleeping partners. He noticed that people who were asleep had regular periods during the night when their eyes moved rapidly. With a co-worker, Nathaniel Kleitman, he investigated this further. Not only did they find that this was a universal occurrence, but they made the fascinating discovery that people woken during one of these periods of Rapid Eye Movement (REM) were far more likely to report dreams.

Since that time sleep has been analyzed more and more, using increasingly sophisticated sleep laboratories. A standard language for describing different levels of sleep has evolved, and sleep is now considered to take two main forms—orthodox and REM. Orthodox sleep is itself divided into four stages, and the sequence of these is common to everyone, although there are subtle differences between the very young child and the adult. Most people follow a regular sequence through the various phases of sleep about once every 90 minutes during the night.

Before sleep itself most people drift through a pleasantly relaxed stage where they are half-asleep and half-awake. Their eyes may be closed, but they are daydreaming. The muscles are relaxed, and perception of the outside world gradually gets less. The EEG at this time shows an even rhythm known as alpha waves. This same pattern also occurs when people are meditating, or doing yoga or other similar relaxation techniques. Just before dropping off to sleep people often experience a sudden jumping sensation known as a myoclonic jerk. You seem to be almost asleep, and then your heart suddenly seems to skip a beat and your body jerks in a sudden spasm. At times it can even feel as if you have fallen suddenly, even though you are lying perfectly still.

It is now that the body enters the first real phase of sleep. In Stage 1 the muscles become more relaxed, and the pulse and breathing tend to slow down and become even more regular.

Occasionally, half-remembered thoughts will pass into conscious-ness, and then float out again. In this stage, people are easily woken and will almost certainly deny having slept at all. The EEG during Stage 1 shows small irregular and rapidly changing waves. This is the shallowest stage of sleep, and one in which a person can be extremely responsive to outside disturbance, like the crying of a child.

You may have found that on those occasions when your own children are asleep you can sometimes go into their room and see them wake at the slightest noise; at other times it takes far more to rouse them, and you may close drawers, pick up the day's toys, and even accidentally drop things, without the children stirring at all. These differences are explained by the fact that the children are at a different stage of sleep.

In adults the full sleep cycle—the ultradian rhythm—takes approximately 90 to 100 minutes. In babies the cycle is much shorter, being only about 50 minutes. In other words, babies tend to sleep in multiples of 50 rather than 90 minutes, and after a feeding may sleep for about 100, 150 or 200 minutes before waking again. This more rapid turnover of the sleep cycle ex-plains why children are more prone to night-waking than adults.

Stage 1 is not the only level of sleep from which one can fairly easily be woken, but during the next two stages of sleep the sleeper sinks deeper and deeper away from consciousness. In Stage 2 the eyes will not see or register if they are opened, although occasional thoughts may drift through the mind. The EEG shows gradually enlarging waves, which become very slow and large by Stage 3. In alpha waves, when one is drifting off to sleep, there are up to 12 waves per second. By Stage 3 there is only one each second. The mind is much less responsive, even though one may be woken by fairly quiet sounds during Stage 2.

By Stage 3, it takes a much louder noise to awaken a sleeper. People who are deliberately woken up during this phase of sleeping can rarely recall anything, and all the bodily functions continue to slow right down. Muscles are relaxed, the tempera-ture drops, and even the blood pressure slowly falls.

However, the deepest sleep is experienced during Stage 4

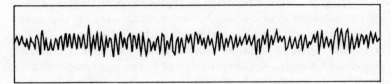

Awake

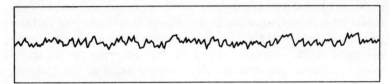

Stage 1 sleep (Shallow sleep)

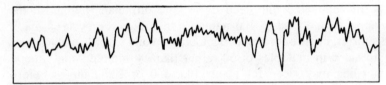

Stage 2 sleep (Gradually enlarging waves)

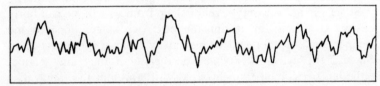

Stage 3 sleep (Mostly large slow waves)

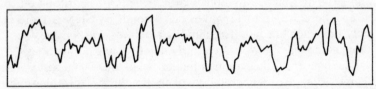

Stage 4 sleep (All large slow waves)

The diagrams show sections from an EEG print-out. The brain-wave patterns show four different levels of sleep.

sleep. This phase is also sometimes called the delta stage after the very large slow delta waves recorded on the EEG.

During this phase there is virtually total oblivion. Dreams are only very rarely recalled from this stage, although sleepwalking and bedwetting may begin. It is very difficult to awaken someone from this depth of sleep, although parents often retain a curious, specific sensitivity for the noise of crying, even at this stage of the night. It is almost as if the mind can remain focused and on the lookout for certain very specific noises. I remember well countless occasions when I have gone out to see a patient during the night and found it almost impossible to awaken my wife to tell her where I was going, only to see her wake up almost instantly at the sound of a distressed cry from one of the children. I have yet to find any truly satisfactory explanation for this phenomenon, but it is one that all parents know.

It is interesting and obviously very important to remember that while an adult spends 80% of his sleeping time in deep sleep and 20% in light sleep, babies have a very different ratio with about half their sleeping time being light sleep. With this mismatch of sleeping rhythms it is hardly surprising that problems can and do occur. Hopefully the baby who comes to wakefulness during the night will just turn over and go back to sleep again. If he doesn't, then the parents' sleep pattern will be rudely interrupted.[3]

Having reached Stage 4, after a total period of around 90 minutes, the sleeper will suddenly enter the curious period of REM sleep. The EEG recording changes abruptly, and this crude measurement of brain activity resembles waking more than sleeping. The eyes dart about rapidly, the pulse and breathing may be irregular, and the fingers and toes may twitch and jerk. However, purposeful movements of the limbs, as in walking, are impossible during this stage. A sleeper who is woken during REM sleep will almost always report a dream. This REM period typically lasts for 10–15 minutes, and then the climb down the ladder of the other stages of sleep begins again. All in all, in a good night's sleep, the whole cycle may be repeated four or five times. The average turnover time for the cycle in adults is 90 minutes, in the new-born child it is 47 minutes, and in the three- to-eight-month-old it is 50 minutes. It is very likely that waking is more frequent in children than in adults as children pass into lighter levels of sleep more often during the night, and there are therefore nearly twice as many occasions when they can be woken up easily than there are for adults. Outside noises and other disturbances become a far more important cause of waking for children as they will more often be at a light level of sleep.

It is still difficult to know exactly what is going on during REM sleep. It used to be thought that such occurrences as penile erection and the darting about of the eyes were in response to the content of the dreams, but this is no longer thought to be the case. It seems that these physical changes are not caused by mental activity, but just go on at the same time. What is certain is that the REM stage is essential. If for some reason—say, the use of sleeping tablets—the amount of REM sleep is reduced, there will be a compensatory increase of REM sleep for a while. Experimental work which has deprived people—volunteers, naturally—of certain phases of sleep shows that if the sufferer is deprived of Stage 4 sleep only, he will tend to be lethargic and run down the next day, but if the REM sleep is lost then more complex skills such as learning and memory will be interfered with. It is now known that during the delta phase of sleep the pituitary gland at the base of the brain increases its production of Human Growth Hormone (HGH). This is involved in the general revitalization of tissues and may explain some of the problems experienced if this phase of sleep is lost. This relationship between delta sleep and HGH release does not apply to the first three months of life, but otherwise granny was right. You do grow in your sleep.[4] Nevertheless, the opposite does not hold true. There is certainly no evidence that children who sleep less than average grow less than average.

Sleep research is still in its infancy and much remains to be understood. However, before we leave this complex area it is intriguing to note that the typical sleep cycle not only applies to all humans; it applies to reptiles, to birds, and to all mammals with one exception. Why the spiny anteater does not have REM sleep I cannot imagine. Perhaps it has nothing worth dreaming about.

This analysis of the different levels of sleep is only one way of looking at the subject. Another way is to measure the total lengths of time that people sleep, and here one runs into all manner of new problems.

Perhaps the trickiest one to solve is the fact that people are extremely poor at estimating how long they sleep. Insomniacs who claim, and honestly believe, that they hardly sleep a wink have on occasion been studied in hospital sleep laboratories. Both observations and EEG studies show that such people may sleep as long and as deeply as their non-insomniac friends, even though the subject still believes that the night during which he was studied was a poor one.

There is no doubt that some people do need more sleep than others. There are many people who cope well with only a few hours of sleep each night, and others who feel shattered without at least nine or ten. There is hardly a truly great person in history who is not said to have been a short sleeper. Every major emperor and every wartime leader is reported to have managed on only three or four hours of sleep a night. Napoleon, Winston Churchill and Eleanor Roosevelt are all reputed to have been refreshed by a brief nap during a crisis.

I somehow doubt it. To be considered dynamic and somehow above sleeping is not something that the far-from-modest people who become leaders are likely to deny, and the near universality of the myth makes me more sceptical still. I am sure that such men and women are not dullards who doze their lives away, but I would be far more convinced if better evidence were forthcoming about their sleeping habits.

A few years ago a sleep research laboratory looked at the difference between long and short sleepers.[5] To summarize their extensive findings, they found that people who apparently required less than average sleep were effective, practical people, such as top business executives, applied scientists, and political leaders; the long sleepers were found to be less conventional and more creative people, and generally more critical in their social and political views.

This is a splendid piece of research. Whether you are a short or a long sleeper you end up praised. Either you are dynamic or creative. You can pride yourself in being unconventional, or equally in being a leader of men. No one can complain, however they are described.

Whatever type of sleeper you are, you will inevitably run into problems if you do not get enough sleep—enough for your needs. Sleep deprivation can be very serious. I have stressed that the majority of children who wake at night rarely suffer as a result. If they are tired they will usually make up their sleep requirements at other times of the day. If a two-year-old is tired there is nothing to stop him having a sleep at any time he wants; if an adult is tired, housework, or an outside job often makes that impossible. A parent may be on the go all day. It becomes most important that he or she gets enough sleep at night, and a wakeful child in the early hours will certainly prevent this. The child may have had enough sleep, or will catch up later. The parent does not get a chance.

Occasional sleepless nights are not too bad. After a parent has sat up all night with an infrequent sleepless child, for example one who has an ear infection, he or she may feel physically exhausted, but at least there is the consolation that the next night will almost certainly be restful. When a child wakes repeatedly, night after night, week after week, the feelings are quite different. It is now realized that disturbed sleep, even though it may add up to eight or more hours in a night, produces more tiredness than six hours of undisturbed sleep. This important fact will be looked at again in Chapter 14 when we look at survival techniques for the parents of sleepless children.

For centuries sleep deprivation has been used as a highly effective method of torture. Prisoners who could withstand floggings and other physical punishments would regularly be reduced to useless wrecks when their sleep was deprived night after night. Today's sleepless parents know just how they felt! Observation of people who have been kept awake for prolonged periods show that they pass through several stages. Initially there is irritability and anger, followed by difficulty in paying attention, and finally hallucinations. Few parents ever reach this last stage, but the others are well known.

One of the best known cases of sleep deprivation in recent years was the New York disc jockey, Peter Tripp, who stayed awake for 200 hours for charity. Throughout the whole period he kept broadcasting, and was also under assessment by medical researchers. To start with he did well, but then the hallucinations set in. At one stage he ran down the hallway attempting to escape from the doctors. He had become quite convinced that they were undertakers who had come to bury him. Following the "wakathon" he became pretty seriously depressed for some time, but despite this, after a single really good night's sleep he began to function remarkably well. In chronically sleep-deprived people this depression may be far more longlasting.

Peter Tripp, for all his adventures, is not the world record holder for sleeplessness. This dubious distinction is held at the time of writing by Mrs. Maureen Weston of Cambridgeshire, England. She stayed awake in a rocking chair marathon for 18 days and 17 hours, but according to the *Guinness Book of Records* suffered no lasting ill-effects despite some hallucinations toward the end. Parents of sleepless children must feel that people who keep themselves awake deliberately and voluntarily must be completely crazy. Sleep is too precious. Modern research has shown that it is also infinitely more valuable and complicated than people had ever before realized. It is hardly surprising that sleepless nights cause parents such despair.

The Sleepless Child— Why Problems Arise

"Why does it happen?"
"What have I done to deserve all this trouble?"
"Is it my fault?"
"Where did I go wrong?"

Almost every letter that I received from the parents of sleepless children asked the same basic questions. What everyone wants to know is why *they* should be suffering when their friends and neighbors are not. These parents rarely had any satisfaction in their inquiries. One mother who had seen family doctors, pediatricians and social workers with her two exhausting children wrote, "I can honestly say that no one has come up with a convincing reason why they should be bad sleepers."

Without a doubt the most common explanation put forward for sleep disturbance is that the whole problem is the fault of the parents. Many doctors, nurses, grandparents, neighbors and friends have no second thoughts about making this point. As one mother wrote to me, expressing an opinion that turned up over and over again, "The one thing I feel strongly about is that doctors are exceptionally good at making parents feel totally to blame because their children don't do what the books say they should. My doctor was always telling me that all I needed was firmness—with the result that I felt like a weak-willed, ineffectual drip. I was very relieved when my second child proved to be so 'good' and I was reassured that I wasn't turning my children into self-willed monsters because of my inefficient parenting."

One well-respected medical journal which carried an otherwise excellent article on this problem included the sentence, "Many sleep problems originate from the way the baby is managed, or mismanaged, in early childhood, and bad habit formation is one of the most common causes of trouble in sleep."[1] I remain convinced that this is only a major factor in a minority of cases.

All children are sleepless at times, and this next chapter looks at some of the simple common causes of childhood sleeplessness and shows how a parent's reaction may prolong what would have otherwise been a temporary problem. You may find that your particular problem can be traced back to a specific episode, like an earache—and it is certainly vital to consider this possibility— but there are nevertheless a huge number of parents for whom this will not apply. Certainly I do not want to give the impression that if you cannot sort out your problems in this way then the problem must be your fault. This attitude has frequently been displayed by doctors. One eminent pediatrician wrote in 1922 that "a sleepless baby is a reproach to his guardians."[2] And a very recent article stated that, "The unhappy insecure infant presents the greatest problems over a long period. He may cry when first put to bed and wake at intervals throughout the night demanding attention."[3] Is it any wonder that parents become distressed? Wakefulness appears to occur because either they mishandle the situation or because their children are "unhappy and insecure."

I am far less certain. There is no doubt that parents can sometimes greatly aggravate the problem, but very frequently it is entirely out of their hands. The possible causes can be looked at in two groups. There are the factors that cause the problem in the first place, and those that keep a pre-existing problem going. There are also a huge number of occasions when it is simply impossible to pin down a particular cause, and even more when it is of no value to do so. Understanding may add satisfaction, but it doesn't always add sleep!

It cannot be stressed too often that children are only seen as having sleep problems when the parents suffer. There is a huge cultural element to this. For example, in Europe children traditionally stay up late to have an evening meal with their parents. American families on vacation and eating in American restaurants often look on with amazement at four- and five-year-old children joining their parents, the restaurant owners, for a full family meal at 11 o'clock at night when business is over. The children may well have had a nap, or at least a rest, early in the evening and will almost certainly sleep well after finishing their five-course dinner. To a certain extent, therefore, one of the causes of sleep problems is the society and culture in which the child lives. Societies in which the children traditionally sleep with their parents have far fewer sleep problems. For a number of reasons, which I will look at in Chapter 10, this is not seen as the norm in many Western societies. Yet again, the attitude of society may be very much responsible for the existence of the problem in that it molds parental attitudes and actions.

A great deal of the research that has gone on into the causes of sleep problems runs completely against the old opinion that sleep disorders are the parents' fault. One particularly impressive study on children from birth to school age noted that sleeping and feeding difficulties were probably the most frequent topics on which advice is sought from health care professionals.[4,5] In a summary of their findings the authors said, "Our results suggest that some of the advice that comes from these sources is not always very helpful and may have little real experience behind it." They go on to say that the result of research into such everyday problems "has not filtered through very effectively to those who need it." The sort of comments I quoted earlier in this chapter would appear to confirm this.

The authors of the study, Martin Richards and Judith Bernal, had been taking a detailed but broad look at the development of about 100 children, and when they found that at 14 months the

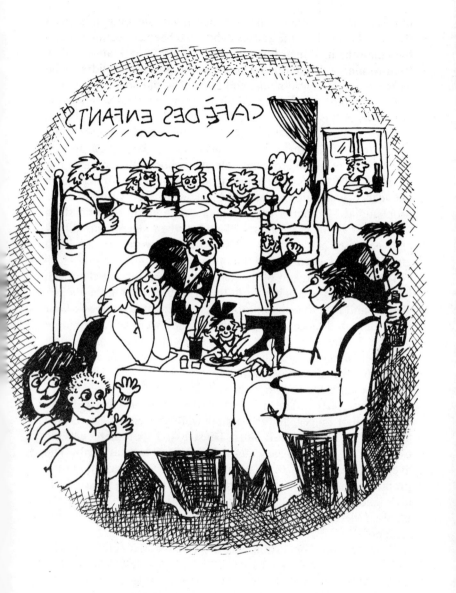

most common problem causing concern was sleeping difficulties they tried to analyze the causes. They had been collecting data on the children since their birth and had plenty to look at, and they tried to pinpoint differences between the group of children who were seen to have problems, and those who did not.

To begin with they analyzed birth order, sex, and whether the child was bottle or breast fed. There was no difference between the two groups. Then they looked at their earlier records and found that at all the earlier interviews—at 8, 14, 20 and 30 weeks—the problem group was sleeping shorter than others. For example, at 8 weeks the longest period of uninterrupted sleep between 6 P.M. and 6 A.M. for those who were going to have problems at 14 months was 5.6 hours. The group with no sleep problems averaged 8.8 hours of undisturbed sleep. This difference persisted at each age assessed. In other words, the problem group always lagged behind the others.

This was not the end of it. Their figures were detailed enough for them to analyze behavior in the first 10 days of a child's life. They found that the sleep problem group spent less time in their cribs and cried more. It appeared that they were generally more irritable babies—an opinion confirmed by the results of a neurological examination and sucking test that had been carried out on the eighth and ninth days of life.

They then went back further still and analyzed the records of the babies' births. The mothers of the sleep problem children were in labor longer, and the infants were slower to begin crying and regular breathing. It must be stressed that there was no evidence of any damage caused by oxygen lack at birth. The average time from birth to the first cry was 36.4 seconds in the problem group, and 19.6 seconds in the others. These are averages and all children by no means fit this pattern. Both my children were quick deliveries and early criers, and yet dreadful sleepers.

However, the conclusion was inescapable. The children who had sleep problems at 14 months had probably always had problems and had been more fussy and irritable as early as the first 10 days of life. If this is the case it seems extremely unlikely that parental mishandling is to blame.

For years the parents of sleepless children have been told that they have problems because of the way in which they care for their children. In fact, the way that they care is frequently a response to the problem, and not the cause of it. A desperate mother will do almost anything to try and help, and then has to listen while others tell her that what she does is the reason for her problems. As Richards and Bernal concluded, "The parents of the problem babies used a wider range of tactics to deal with night-waking. This is hardly surprising, as our results showed that there is no obvious cure and so parents are likely to work through all possible remedies."

This research is not unique. A study in 1957 looked at 200 children and found no correlation between sleep problems and birth weight, nor weight gain. It did find a correlation with mild asphyxia at birth.[6] This finding had also been used by other earlier researchers, and twenty-four years later another article in the same journal stated that most studies, but not all, found an association between wakefulness and perinatal adversity, and early restlessness or high activity."[7]

Another study disputed these findings. A group of sleep problem children were compared with a group of controls and no correlation between birth history and subsequent sleeping problems was found.[8] Admirable although the study is, I have reservations as to how the groups were chosen. The researchers involved were asked to provide names of children with sleep problems, and an equal number of children the same age were chosen as controls. It turned out that a third of the parents of the control group said that their children had sleep problems. It was only because this had not come to the researchers notice that they were not included in the problem group. There are bound to be immense difficulties interpreting results when this sort of thing happens.

Whether the problem starts at birth or slightly afterwards, there seems little doubt that some children sleep badly whatever their parents might do. There is also no doubt that some children develop their problems later. It is probably fair to conclude that many problems are the result of the infant's behavior and individuality, while others result from the parents' behavior. Obviously there is little that you can do about the characteristics that your child was born with, although you can learn to cope with the problems they cause. However, when the chief cause has been parental there is much more that you can do.

Simple causes of sleep-upsets happen to every child, and yet on occasion they can be the acorn from which grows the oak of persistent sleepless nights. Even the rebelliousness that is normal for all toddlers can cause long-term problems. The previously normally sleeping child may one night call out that he wants a drink. He may be given it, and ten minutes later calls out to be taken to the bathroom. Another request for a drink follows. . . . The parents' response to all this is vitally important. If, after each and every request, the child gets a kiss, a cuddle, even a nursery rhyme or short story, what incentive is there for him to stay alone in his crib?

All manner of evidence has been presented to suggest that this desire for attention, along with the way that parents react to it, is the major factor in sleep disturbance. This is apparently confirmed by the fact that sleepless children are often reported to sleep better in a hospital. This is hardly proof. A busy nurse with a ward full of children is much less likely to know that a child is awake than a mother in a small home. The fact that a child is not *known* to be awake is not proof that he is asleep!

One study of two-year-olds made the observation that only 3.3% of those in residential nurseries had sleep problems compared with 37% of those at home.[9] This had been taken as proof that parents cause sleep problems. Again, it may simply be that the nursery staff did not notice. Another study examined the different ways that two nurses looked after babies in a nursery. One nurse tended to respond more quickly to crying, and with this nurse the children tended to cry more often. It is tempting to conclude that her quicker speed of response encouraged the children to have more sleep problems. However, it was also noted that the slower responding nurse was more skilled at soothing the children.[10] These things are never simple, and to sift out the different causes for a complex problem like sleeplessness is extraordinarily difficult.

A final observation that adds considerable weight to the conclusion that sleepless children need not be the parents' fault is the fact that one child in a family can have dreadful sleep problems while the other does not. Sometimes the first child has the problem, and sometimes the later children. Very many parents wrote to me insisting that although they had brought up their children identically, one had slept perfectly and the other very poorly. This can even apply to twins. I have records of a number of twins where one slept much better than the other. Some of the parents found that when one twin cried persistently at night as a baby, putting him in with the sleeping twin had a calming effect. One might think that this would have the opposite effect, but according to a parents of twins association this usually does not occur. If you have twins with a sleeping problem, it may well be worth taking note of this curious observation.

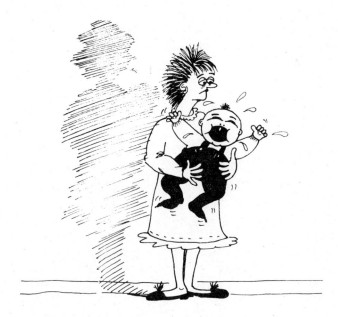

PROBLEMS
AND
SOME SOLUTIONS

• 4 •

Simple Sleep Problems

Not all the sleep problems that parents and children face are as long-term or as distressing as those described in Chapter 1. All children, however well they normally sleep, have occasional disturbed nights for some reason or another. There can hardly be a child in the world who has not kept his parents awake while he was teething, or had some other temporary physical or emotional upset.

Such short-term disturbances may be frustrating and annoying at the time, but they usually settle down. To be able to recognize a cause, and hopefully to do something about it, makes parents feel far less frustrated and angry than when the sleeplessness seems to have come out of the blue. One of the things that makes parents of long-term sleepless children most frustrated is the lack of any discernible reason for their child's apparent distress.

Unfortunately, a simple problem such as teething or colic can be the seed from which a major sleep disturbance may grow. The way that parents react to this is extremely important. If a problem is dealt with effectively, then the child's usual sleep pattern may return. If it is mishandled, then disaster may follow. It is therefore important to consider these simple causes, both for themselves and for the long-term effects that they can sometimes have on the family's sleep. These relatively simple and understandable causes of sleeplessness obviously affect most children at some time or other. Usually the disturbance is temporary. However, there are occasions when it can be the beginning of a more prolonged problem.

Think of Billy, for example. He usually sleeps well, enjoys going to bed, and in every way is a happy, normal three-year-old. One night he wakes with a sore throat from a cold. His mother, quite understandably, takes him from his bed, carries him downstairs to a warm, well-lit living room. The television is on. He's given an aspirin, but is then played with for another half-hour or so. His father may have come home late from work and not have seen him all day. It's the perfect opportunity to cuddle and play.

Eventually the time comes for him to go back to bed. Now if you were Billy and had the choice of lying alone in a cold bed or being downstairs in the heart of a happy family, would you go back to sleep? How the family deals with either Billy's renewed crying, or else his reluctance to go to bed the next night, may have an immense effect on his sleep pattern—and on his parents' sleep too—over the next few months.

Billy has obviously realized that there are better ways of spending the night than lying in a darkened room. Children quickly learn that crying at night either gets them brought downstairs or taken into their parents' bed. It may be that there are occasions when you do not mind this happening.

I well remember one mother whose husband often had to travel abroad on business. When he was away she would always take her child into her bed if he woke up during the night. She admitted that she felt happier that way. However, when her husband was at home she bitterly resented her child's intrusion and could not understand why he kept waking up.

As a first step in trying to more fully understand your own child's sleep problems, there are a number of questions that you should consider. First of all, can you pinpoint the particular occasion when the problem started? What do you do when your child wakes? Are you consistent in how you try to cope with the waking? Put yourself in your child's position and look at your ways of coping through his eyes. What does he get out of waking?

For instance, does he get a hug, a drink, or a play period that he would not normally get? Do you yourself get anything out of the way you deal with the problem, like the mother who occasionally enjoyed having her child sleeping with her? What effect does the repeated waking have on the rest of the family, and does the child get some benefit from this?

In any case of repeated wakefulness, it is important to consider all these points. Sometimes you will be able to spot some aspect of your care that is actually aggravating the situation.

So, what should you do if a child who normally sleeps well wakes in the night? Perhaps the most important thing to remember is that what you do now may give you an easier night tonight, but at the same time may in some way reward your child and so encourage the waking to be repeated.

If such a child wakes up while you are in the middle of watching a film on television, it is very tempting to bring him down with you rather than sit up in his room, possibly missing the most important part of the story. That is fine, provided that you realize that the child will enjoy cuddling downstairs and will expect the same each time he wakes up. It is probably better to suffer some inconvenience now rather than a lot more in the future. The same rule applies if you have friends with you, or on any occasion that the child might prefer to be awake with you rather than alone in his room.

Jenny was a four-year-old who had always slept well, until one Saturday evening. That day she had been catching a cold, and at about 10 o'clock she woke up with an earache. Her parents had invited friends around for dinner—friends who hadn't seen Jenny since she was a few weeks old. Denise, her mother, didn't want to break up the party and brought her down for a cuddle. Jenny found herself the center of attraction and reveled in the attention. Someone gave her an after-dinner mint. Someone else affectionately bounced her up and down on his knee. Everyone enjoyed playing with her.

The next night Jenny would not go to sleep. Every time that Denise left her she cried and screamed, demanding to be taken downstairs. Obviously she expected the same fun as the night before. She made such a commotion that eventually she was taken downstairs and cuddled, where—even though there was no dinner party going on—there was warmth and music and company.

This was one of those relatively rare occasions where the only answer would have been to have persevered in leaving her in her room. For the average long-term sleepless child this approach usually fails, but when it is apparent that the child has got into a habit of wanting to be taken from his room as he expects some form of reward, then it may succeed. Denise had several terrible, almost unbearable evenings with Jenny, insisting that she could not go downstairs until eventually the message sank in and sleep returned.

Please remember that I am not saying that you should *never* take a child from his room. But it is certainly worth keeping such trips as short and as unexciting as possible. A thirsty child who calls for a drink should be given one drink and then left again. If the drink is followed by a story, lullaby or cuddle, then no one can be surprised if the moment the door is closed the child calls out for another drink. Similarly, many of the common, simple sleep problem causes that we will now consider need dealing with kindly and effectively and always with one eye open to future implications.

I cannot stress enough that these suggestions only apply to those parents who believe that they have a problem. If you enjoy your child being with you all evening, then that is fine and you will have no concern if such waking spells occur.

THE SLEEPING ENVIRONMENT

Perhaps the simplest of the simple causes of sleep problems are connected with the child's sleeping environment. After all, if you are expecting your child to be happy spending a sizeable proportion of his life in his bedroom, then it should obviously be a pleasant and happy place. In particular you should avoid using the bedroom as a threat. If you tell the child who misbehaves to go to his room as a punishment, then you cannot be surprised if he doesn't want to go there at bedtime.

Decorations

If you child is old enough, try to involve him in choosing decorations for the room, whether it be pictures, posters or wallpaper. You may naturally wish to retain editorial control, particularly if faced with a demand to have one wall pink, one orange, and the ceiling purple. You may find that a certain decoration will need changing: a pattern on a curtain that looks charming by daylight may appear as a ravenous monster when the moon shines through it at night. If your child is frightened of the room, it is certainly worth exploring such possible causes.

Lighting

Lighting can be very important. An older child usually likes lighting that he can control himself, possibly at his bedside. Many children are frightened of the dark, and it is likely that this is something they are taught by their parents. That is not as odd as it sounds. If a baby wakes and cries at night, his mother will almost certainly come to him, and as she comes through the door she will put the light on. As she leaves she will put the light out. Light becomes associated with comfort and company. Darkness becomes linked with loneliness. If there is any practical way you can avoid your child becoming conditioned like this, then try to do so. Do not put the light on, at least not the main light, if you can possibly manage without it.

Children who are frightened of the dark are often comforted by a very low wattage night light. Better yet is a dimmer switch on the main light. Each night the lighting can be set slightly lower, almost without the child realizing that there is a change.

Obviously, you cannot manipulate the moonlight quite so easily, though you can vary the thickness of curtains. You might think that such seasonal matters as temperature or time of night might affect sleeping habits, but a survey of two hundred children

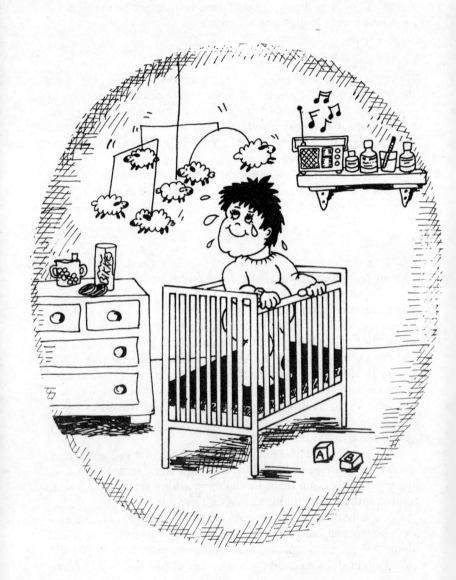

in 1957 found that seasonal differences of light and temperature showed no relationship with sleep problems at the age of three months, babies born at different times of year having problems in equal proportions.[1]

Windows

Among adults the debate as to whether the window should be left open or closed at night can cause heated arguments. Paul Simon's song *You're Kind,* on the *Still Crazy After All These Years* album, even cites such a dispute as a reason for ending a relationship. Nothing is new. In the 1883 edition of the *Homoeopathic Vade Mecum* by E. Harris Ruddock, I found the following opinion. "Airy well-ventilated sleeping apartments should be ranked with the most important requirements of life, both in health and disease. If any person will take the trouble to stand in the sun and look at his own shadow on a white plastered wall, he will easily perceive that his whole body is a smoking mass of corruption with a vapour exhaling from every part of it. This vapour is subtle, acrid, and offensive to the smell. If retained in the body it becomes morbid, but if reabsorbed, highly deleterious. Unpleasant as it is to dwell on such a subject, it is yet true that the exhalations from the human lungs and skin, if retained and undiluted with a continuous supply of oxygen, are the most repulsive with which we can come in contact."

This is a classic case of an unwarranted conclusion being made from an observation. It may not get me quoted in a hundred years, but all I can say is "do what you want." Personally, I like the window open. At the moment, Katy keeps hers shut since a school friend told her that witches will get in if she leaves it open. I don't mind either way.

Noise

An important consideration regarding the room itself is noise. Modern houses and apartments often have very thin walls, and inevitably children can hear what is going on both outside and elsewhere in the house. It is far better for the parents to carry on downstairs normally, rather than trying to keep particularly quiet to let the child get to sleep. In the same way as adults living in a city stop hearing traffic noise that would appear deafening to a country dweller, so do children adapt to ordinary household noise. Think back to your own childhood. Wasn't it much more pleasant being able to hear the murmur of voices and domestic life being carried on downstairs? Some noise may help combat the loneliness your child may feel at bedtime. Children are more likely to be more disturbed by silence rather than by everyday noise, though if you have a disco party in the room under theirs you can expect their reaction to be the same as yours would be if your neighbors tried the same trick.

The bed

As for the bed, all that matters is that the child should find it comfortable. Most babies sleep in a crib, and it is not possible to say exactly when the change to a bed should be made. Perhaps the best time is when it appears that the baby can manage to climb over the sides of the crib. If he can do that, then he would be safer in a bed. It may not be easy keeping him there, but at least he can't break anything falling out, which can happen with children climbing from cribs. Be sure that any crib you use is safe. The bars of the crib should not be more than about three inches apart, as it has been known for a child to die with his head wedged through a wider gap. It is also worth checking that there are no screws or bolts that clothing can hook on to, as these can cause strangulation.

It all sounds rather gruesome, but bedtime isn't usually that dangerous! Once a child has graduated to a bed, then the design and bedding are up to you.

Bedding and warmth

It is important that babies and children are warm enough in bed. A child who kicks and wriggles his way from under his blankets and then gets cold in a chilly bedroom is bound to wake up. Preventing coldness is an easy way to avoid one cause of wakefulness. The bedroom itself should be pleasantly warm, particularly for the very young, but do make sure that it does not become increasingly hot during the evening. It may be worth fitting a separate thermostat to any radiator in the child's room to ensure that the temperature stays reasonably constant.

The actual design of bedding often does not matter. However, the child who always seems to end up on top of his bedding may be better off in a sleeping bag. These bags are not a good idea for the first few weeks of life, as the newborn baby prefers to be wrapped snugly in a blanket, but after that a sleeping bag, or footed-pajamas, can prevent small children from getting too cold. Always make sure that you choose one that is large enough. As an alternative way to stop the restless child from getting too cold, blanket clips come in handy.

Pillows are best avoided in the first year as there is at least a theoretical risk of suffocation. Later, pillow design and texture is a matter of personal taste.

Boredom and loneliness

Always remember that your child may find his bedroom a boring place. An adequate bedtime supply of toys, books, mobiles, or activity centers may make that period between your saying good night and your child going to sleep much less of a strain—and may keep him occupied if he is an early-riser.

In addition, your child may not only be bored but also lonely. If you have two children, you may find that they sleep better in the same room than apart. As one mother wrote me, "Someone advised us to put Paul, the non-sleeping one, in with his sister. We thought this was crazy, and would lead to Paul waking her up as well, and giving us double the trouble. In fact we gave it a chance and the opposite happened." Twins can be helped in the same way, and it is certainly a solution well worth giving a try.

Drinks and potties

As far as the rest of the bedroom is concerned there are a few other simple points worth considering. The problem of the child who regularly wakes up because of thirst may be helped by leaving a glass of water on a bedside table. There is no evidence that giving a child a drink at bedtime or during the night makes bed-wetting more likely (see Chapter 8). Such a simple move may often prevent the child from calling out. In a similar way, you may avoid being disturbed by the older child who calls to be taken to the bathroom if you leave a potty by his bed.

EMOTIONAL PROBLEMS

In adults, sleepless nights are more often caused by emotional problems than physical ones, and such causes can be extremely important for children—even very young ones. A parent in the hospital, the first week at a new school, a new baby in the family, the death of a pet, even the happy excitement that comes before Christmas—all these events can upset the naturally relaxed sleep of a child. Understanding why your child is worried, talking with him, reassuring and explaining can all help.

Sarah's parents eventually realized this. Sarah was six and began to sleep badly when her baby brother was born. Every night was the same. She would lie awake sobbing, and her parents became distraught. They were certain that she must be jealous, and every day they would stress to her over and over again how much they loved her. But it did not seem to help.

They tried discussing it with her, cuddling her, buying her little presents, but all to no avail. Then Sarah's schoolteacher gave them the clue they were looking for. Sarah had painted a picture at school of a soldier with a sword. When asked who it was, she replied that "It is the soldier that kills baby boys." Gradually the story came together. Shortly before her brother's birth Sarah had heard the Bible story about King Herod putting to death all the male babies in an attempt to kill the infant Jesus. Sarah, like all six-year-olds, had no real concept of history. She was convinced that her brother was going to be killed. Far from being jealous, she loved him intensely, and the more her parents had been especially kind to her, the more she became convinced that they were making up for the fact that he would soon be dead. Once she was reassured by them that this was not the case, her sleep pattern reverted to normal.

Such emotional factors as these can be important from a very young age, as even tiny infants react to parental stress and to changes in the family atmosphere. A particularly awkward vicious cycle can then be set up in which a child becomes aware that his parent is under stress, and the child sleeps badly, thus increasing the parent's stress. Such a chain can spiral to heights of desperation in a very short time.

THE OVERTIRED CHILD

The child who has had a very active and exciting day may sometimes seem to be too tired to sleep. It is certainly a feeling that I have experienced. Despite being physically exhausted, sleep will just not come. This is probably more a failure to unwind properly than anything else, but it can be a self-perpetuating problem in the sleepless child. Ways of preparing a child for sleep are dealt with in the next chapter.

HUNGER

It is rarely a problem with older children, but hunger is very often blamed as being the reason for wakefulness in babies. Most mothers whose babies wake at night will respond, quite naturally, by feeding them. The fact that the baby takes the feeding cannot be taken as absolute proof that it was hunger that woke him.

It is traditionally believed that the well-fed baby with a full stomach will sleep deeply and peacefully until he needs his next feeding, but this has been shown not always to be the case. Some underfed babies sleep longer than some very well-fed ones, and the link between feeding and sleeping is not quite as close as many people think.

This would not matter if this particular traditional belief did not affect the mother's management of her child. A mother who has been brought up to feel that adequate feeding makes a child sleep is bound to reach the reverse conclusion that a child who does not sleep is underfed. As a result, all manner of extra feedings may be given in an attempt to correct what is seen as underfeeding. The child who is waking because of teething, colic, or loneliness is then simply given extra milk—often thickened with cereal. The result may be a child who not only is teething, colicy, lonely and awake, but is also fat. The results of such overfeeding are only too apparent.

The normal feeding pattern of a young baby thus means that to begin with night feedings is inevitable. Thankfully these can gradually be stopped, but many mothers see giving up the night feeding as an achievement, a sign that the child is making progress. As a result if the baby starts waking when the feeding has been stopped the mothers are very reluctant to give it again, seeing it as a backward step and something to be ashamed of.

It is far better to realize that it is not a failure and to gradually adjust the baby's feeding times to your own more sociable hours. For instance, if a baby regularly wakes at one in the morning for a feeding, it might be better to pre-empt this by waking him for a feeding when you go to bed. He'll get his food. You'll feel much better. You certainly won't be waking up from the depths of a very deep sleep. He won't come to any harm, and moreover, you won't either. If he wakes a little earlier in the morning as a result, that's a lot better than waking in the middle of the night. It is certainly well worth a try, even if it does not always succeed.

With the older child hunger is rarely a problem, and if it does occur it is obviously much easier to deal with.

FOOD

The link between different types of food and the quality of sleep is much debated. All sorts of different foods are reputed to help or hinder sleep, and most of the suggestions owe more to custom and tradition than to science. For instance, cheese is said to cause more vivid dreams, but as everyone dreams every night, and "vivid" is a difficult quality to measure, it is very hard to be certain.

A study in 1934 looked into the link between different foods and sleep in children and concluded that the food eaten at the last meal before retiring does have a marked effect on the quality of sleep.[2] In particular, they found that hard-to-digest foods—defined as slowly digested foods which can tend to cause flatulence—lead to more disturbed nights than if the child has had its normal supper! Unfortunately, the normal supper was not defined. However both the hard-to-digest foods and the "normal" supper resulted in more disturbed nights than a light supper of cornflakes and milk. I cannot help but wonder if this is not simply the known effect of milk in helping sleep.

Much of the advice available on feeding children comes from advertisers and tends to be biased. The timing of the last meal is generally unimportant; babies often settle down immediately after a feeding, but in older children the routine of washing, reading stories, watching television and so on usually comes between the evening meal and bedtime. There are no advantages in having a snack at the actual time of retiring, and if anything is eaten it is very important that the teeth are thoroughly brushed.

One potentially extremely important piece of research has recently been reported on the link between diet and sleep patterns in the newborn.[3] In this, 20 healthy children aged 2 to 3 days old were randomly assigned to receive a feeding containing tryptophan in 10% glucose, or valine in 5% glucose. I discuss the effect of the amino acid tryptophan on page 90; valine is also an amino acid, but one which competes with tryptophan for entry into the brain.

The sleep patterns for 3 hours after the feeding were compared with those after a feeding of a routine milk preparation (Similac, an infant formula). The infants fed tryptophan entered active sleep 14.1 minutes sooner than they did after Similac, and entered quiet sleep 39 minutes later. Such observations may not yet sleep 15.8 minutes later than they did after Similac, and entered into quiet sleep 39 minutes later. Such observations may not yet be of any great practical value, but they do confirm that diet does have a scientifically measurable effect on sleep in the newborn.

Many parents have reported that their children are more restless after they have eaten foods containing sugar, though as yet I have no scientific evidence that this is the case. It is certainly worth bearing in mind, and it may be worth noting if any other foods seem to lead to an upset night. I will, however, be returning to one other potentially important aspect of foodstuffs in Chapter 9 when I consider the effects of food additives on sleep, particularly in the hyperactive.

As for bedtime drinks, there is little doubt that milk or water are preferable to fruit juices—if only for the sake of the teeth. Milk does seem to have a helpful effect. (See bedtime routine, page 89.)

WIND

When a baby cries, his mother will eventually pick him up, and as she cuddles him he may burp. The reason for his crying seems very clear: he was in pain because of his gas and the burp helped to relieve this pain.

It may sound obvious put like that, but consider it another way. A crying baby may swallow a lot of air in the act of howling and screaming. When he is picked up, he is held in an upright position which makes it easier for the swallowed air to be released in a burp. He may have been crying because he was cold or bored, and the wind may have been the result, not the cause, of his crying.

In many countries there is no word for this sort of "wind." Certainly no effort is made to ensure that the child brings up his wind after a feeding, something that many Western parents feel is essential. There is no doubt that babies do have wind, but doctors are agreed that far too many symptoms are unjustifiably blamed on it. Try not to assume automatically that because your child burps that wind was the reason he was crying.

Many people think that wind is gas that is formed somewhere in the baby's stomach. In fact, the wind is only the air that has been swallowed. Babies who bring up a lot of wind after a feeding are the ones who have swallowed a lot of air during it. The opposite follows: if your child does not burp after a feed, it simply means that he did not swallow that much air.

The best way to deal with wind is to attempt to prevent it by ensuring that your baby swallows less air during a feeding. With bottle-fed babies you may find that enlarging the hole in the nipple helps, and breast feeding mothers sometimes find that expressing a little milk first does the trick. Pediatricians and child care books all have plenty of advice. Wind is not an important *cause* of sleepless nights; it cannot spontaneously appear during the night and wake a child up, even though a crying child—crying for some other reason—may burp when picked up.

COLIC

Colic is a fascinating condition, not least because of the controversy among many medical experts over whether it exists or not.

At first glance it seems odd that there should be such a controversy at all. Even though no one has a totally convincing explanation, colic affects otherwise perfectly healthy babies in the first few months of life. It consists of periodic attacks of piercing screaming, apparently caused by considerable pain, usually occurring in the evening and associated with drawing up the legs, loud rumblings from the abdomen and a lot of wind passing through the anus. Typically, it always gets better by three to four months. In one study of infants, 54% had stopped having attacks by 2 months, 85% by 3 months, and 100% by 4 months.[4]

Why should there be any dispute about it? It sounds like a fairly clear-cut condition, even if no one knows what causes it. As child care expert Dr. Hugh Jolly has often pointed out, all babies draw up their legs when they cry, and by drawing up their legs are bound to pass wind. Dr. Jolly, and other doctors, feel that the term colic is used far too often. Crying in the evenings may occur because babies sense the excitement in the home on the arrival of the father. Indeed, by six o'clock the baby may simply be bored and scream because he wants company and wants to be played with. Doctors who support this view say that the wind and the apparent discomfort are caused by, not causes of, the screaming.

I am not so sure. There is no doubt that doctors and parents like to have a label to put on something, such as a cause of crying, and on occasions the label may not be appropriate. Both my children had attacks of screaming regularly in the first three months, and these screams were totally different from the screams they used at other times. They also looked like they were in pain. I don't know if they were, or if Dr. Jolly was right and it was just me as a parent assuming that because they were crying they must have been in pain. However, the screams sounded quite different than a hunger or temper cry. Ronald Illingworth is quite certain that colic exists. In his book, *The Normal Child,* he looks at all the possible causes, and at the scepticism about the subject, and remains quite convinced that the condition is a genuine physical one, probably linked with gas being blocked in loops of the bowel.

One particularly interesting study into this subject was carried out at Rochester Child Health Center, New York.[5] It had been suggested that the likelihood of a child having colic might be affected by the mother's age, social class, baby's birth order, sex, weight gain, type of feeding, or family history of allergy. It turned out that none of these was important. Of all the possible causes suggested, intolerance to cow milk is the most popular at present. The fact that breast-fed babies are equally likely to get colic is explained by the fact that cow milk proteins can enter the breast milk from milk drunk by the mother. It must be said that this evidence is inconclusive. But in those babies in whom colic persists past the usual time, it may be worth trying to exclude cow milk from either mother or baby.[6]

Elsewhere, research has been carried out in an attempt to establish the cause of colic and, in particular, to investigate psychological factors in the mother. No connection has been found between emotional problems in mothers and colic in babies. Indeed, one of the few positive results indicates that colic is somewhat more common in the babies of mothers of superior intelligence.

What most convinces me that colic is a separate condition is the impressive response to one particular medication. Ronald Illingworth even goes so far as to say that if the treatment doesn't work then the diagnosis is wrong. Dicyclomine Hydrochloride (marketed in the U.S. as Bentyl and Pasmin, available by prescription only) is a drug that relaxes smooth muscles—the muscle which lines the intestines. I have often seen this drug work within a couple of days where all other treatments have failed, and therefore find it hard to accept Dr. Jolly's view that it is the giving of any medicine that helps to relax the parents' anxiety, rather than a particular effect of this drug.

Mine is not an isolated impression. At least two well-conducted double-blind trials have thoroughly investigated dicyclomine's use in treating colic.[7,8] In thise, parents were given either the drug or an identical-looking and -smelling inactive syrup to administer to their child. Neither parent nor doctor knew until after the results had been recorded which one was the active drug. In both trials the dicyclomine was significantly better at curing the symptoms. This must add weight to the evidence that points to colic's being a physical illness, even if no one can be sure what causes it.

TEETHING

Mark Twain once commented that the great advantage Adam and Eve had over all who followed them was that they avoided teething. There are cynics who say that teething produces nothing but teeth. But it can also cause pain, crying, restlessness, and drooling as well. Many parents blame teething for conditions such as bronchitis, fevers and even convulsions, but there is no doubt at all that teething is not the cause. While these conditions may occur *when* a child is teething, they do not happen *because* of the teething. All doctors have seen serious illnesses that have been delayed in being brought to them because the parents blamed the teeth.

Teething causes its main problems during the time that the first four molars are coming through, usually between a year and eighteen months. This is the stage when teething is most likely to awaken the child. It has been suggested however that teething pains can cause distress to infants as early as the third month, when the points of the teeth begin to stretch and finally break through the tissues lining the outside of the jawbone.[9]

Whenever it occurs, the important question is what can you do about it? In ancient times various substances such as hare's brain, honey and salt mixtures, and hen's grease were used,[10] and Pliny was recorded to have performed an incision of the gums in 23 A.D. These days there are a number of more pleasant treatments. Many parents apply various gels to the sore gums, although thankfully the old mercury teething powders have by now been discarded.

There are gels containing local anesthetics such as benzocaine, but although these work very quickly, the effect does not last long. One trial found that teething gels were effective and found no significant toxic reactions, although it is possible that local sensitization could occur.[11]

Gels are usually applied with a clean fingertip. The massaging effect certainly helps, as massaging may do on its own. Any specially designed hard biscuits for the baby to chew can also help with teething, as may plastic teething rings or other objects. The vital thing about these is to ensure that they are smooth, not thin or brittle, and are a reputable make. Very cheap rings might contain paints with a high lead content.

Chewing helps the teeth erupt, and actual incision is very rarely needed. However, discomfort may often be bad enough to justify a pain-relieving medicine. Medicines should never be used as a matter of routine "just in case," but only if teething is definitely causing pain and restlessness. Numerous different preparations are available. Aspirin is best given as a soluble tablet, and acetaminophen is available in a liquid such as Tylenol. It is essential to follow the dosage instructions accurately, just as you would for an adult drug. Parents are often happy to give an "extra spoonful for luck," which may double the dose of a powerful medication, and this *must* be avoided. In addition, if the child still appears to be in pain despite the medicine, then it is worth getting your doctor to look at him. Your diagnosis of teething may be wrong.

WETNESS AT NIGHT

Children who are still in diapers may be woken up during the night by uncomfortable wetness. Many parents find the solution to this is to use double-layer diapers with a muslin-type one-way diaper liner. The disposable paper one-way liners often used during the day are much less effective. Nowadays many mothers use disposable diapers all the time, but these can become saturated very quickly at night; even the thicker nighttime diapers can still cause problems and it is well worth the addition of an extra absorbent pad inside these for overnight use.

COMMON PAINFUL CONDITIONS

Colic and teething are not the only painful conditions that affect young children. The distress of an earache caused by an ear infection may keep a child awake. So too may tonsilitis, coughs and colds, other similar infections, and even conditions like diaper rash. These conditions are all very common, many perfectly normal children having at least five or six attacks of throat or ear infections in a year. Whatever the cause, it is vitally important to relieve the child's discomfort effectively. With an ear infection, for example, even though your doctor might have provided an antibiotic treatment, it may take some time for this to work, and while you are waiting analgesics like aspirin or acetaminophen can certainly help. If you are in any doubt about whether they can be given along with your doctor's treatment, ask. Similarly, if an attack starts during the night, don't wring your hands until you see the doctor next day. Give pain killers now.

ECZEMA

Many of the parents who wrote to me about their sleepless children told me despairingly of the problems they had with their children who suffered from eczema. This skin condition, which affects about one baby in ten, can cause dreadful itching, and children with eczema often lie awake scratching night after night. The more they scratch, the more they itch. And you know how it is with itches—even trying to ignore them doesn't work. If your child suffers from eczema, antihistamine medicines can be extremely effective. Not only do they stop the itching, but in the right dose they act as sleeping medicines, too. Sleeping medicines are dealt with in detail in Chapter 12 and can be enormously helpful with these children.

Drugs are not the only valuable eczema treatment. It is vital to discuss the condition thoroughly with a doctor and to investigate possible causes, including food allergies. Cow milk, in particular, can sometimes be a triggering factor, and all possibilities need looking into. Self-help groups can also offer much support and advice.

In some children infantile eczema ceases to be a problem after a few months. In others it may go on for several years, usually disappearing by puberty. However, an unfortunate 10% continue to have the problem throughout life.

• 5 •

Bedtime Difficulties

An occasional sleepless night is bearable. The child who lies awake crying with an earache may worry you and certainly tire you. However, when a child either will not go to bed or else wakes repeatedly night after night, week after week, the feelings are quite different.

What becomes overwhelmingly exhausting and debilitating about having a sleepless child is its inevitable persistence. If you can be certain that, even just once a week, you can be guaranteed a restful night, then the anticipation would help keep you going. From both my own experience and that of many correspondents, the thought of having problems night after night is quite depressing. It is this that makes the long-term problems such a torment.

There are several different patterns that long-term sleep problems can take. For a start, there are the difficulties associated with going to sleep in the first place. Then there are those children who repeatedly wake their parents up during the night, and finally there are children who wake their parents up very early in the morning. It is worth considering these one at a time, although many children fit into two, or even three, of the categories.

A survey in 1980 of 124 children whose sleep patterns caused their parents problems found that 35% of the children refused to go to bed before their parents did. As I have already said, the

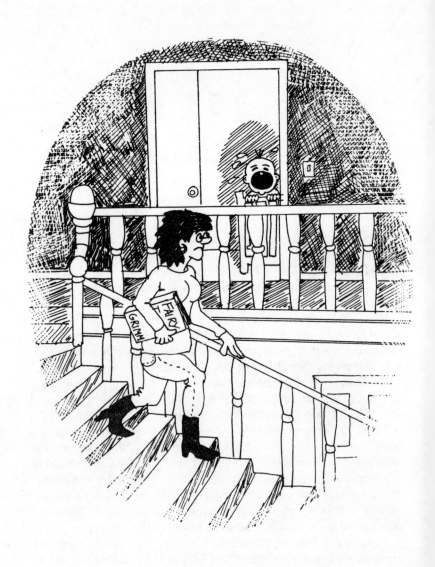

actual time that the child goes to bed does not matter in the least if the parent is happy with the arrangement. What does matter is that parents often like time to themselves in the evenings. The evening is frequently a time to sit and relax, read or watch television, and for parents simply to enjoy one another's company. If one or both parents leave the house during the day to work, then the evening is the only time they can be together. As a result, a screaming child, constant calls for drinks, the patter of tiny feet on the stairs, and the calls of "Mommy, Mommy," can be extremely annoying. If the parents don't mind having the child up with them then the problem disappears, but it is very understandable that for a majority this is not acceptable.

Bedtime problems can take many forms. The child may refuse to go to bed at all and may make noisy objections when he is put there. He may refuse to go with one parent and only go with the other. He may go to bed quite happily, but kick up a terrible fuss when the parent tries to leave, only to settle down again when the parent returns. He may even insist on going through a particular ritual, which may be extremely time consuming, at bedtime. The child may get great security from always following such a ritual.

The whole bedtime routine is discussed in detail later in the chapter, but some of its more aggravating aspects are worth considering now. To the parents' frustration, the child may insist that all the lights are on, or off, that the door is left open at a precise angle, that the window and curtains must be open, or closed, and that certain toys are in exactly the right place. Unless they get completely out of hand, there is no need to discourage these obsessional requests. They may make the child feel more secure.

No, the really maddening child is the one who will not let you leave the room at all without screaming or crying. The traditional advice for dealing with this has always been to "be firm." There are few aspects of the whole problem of sleepless children which cause so much controversy. There are parents and doctors who insist that "being firm" is the only answer. There are others who say that it is never a solution, quoting the findings that I described in Chapter 3 as supporting evidence. You will recall that research showed that sleep problems did not appear to be caused by the way that parents reacted to the child; it seemed more likely that the different parental actions were a response to the sleep difficulties.

As in all controversies like this, there can be little doubt that the truth lies somewhere between the two extremes. Sleep disturbance only matters if it causes a problem for the parents. Some children take a long time getting to sleep; others wake up during the night. It is now obvious that these are no one's fault, but result from all manner of other causes. What does matter is what happens in the house when a child won't settle down or wakes up. In other words, if a child whimpers or cries after you have left him and then rolls over and goes to sleep, there is no problem. However, if, for example, an extremely anxious parent dashes in to see him at the first cry, putting the light on and making a noise in the process, then the child is bound to stay awake and an unnecessary problem will have been created.

For this latter group, and less extreme cases, the "let him cry" approach may work. It has certainly had many advocates in the past. For example, in the 1976 edition of *Baby and Child Care* Dr. Benjamin Spock suggests that if a child whimpers or cries it is wiser to leave him and not go back. He also suggests that the two-year-old who climbs out of his crib at bedtime must be dealt with firmly. He suggests trying a net over the top of cot to stop the child's getting out. He admitted that he was not sure that it was psychologically harmless, but it was at least better than repeated angry scoldings. Spock suggests that after three or four nights of using these approaches the problem will cease even though the child may cry a great deal.

This "crying out" approach certainly works for some babies and children. It can be successful for problems with getting to sleep and with waking up in the night. It is well worth trying, and when it works it is often quick, although for a few nights you will have to put up with varying degrees of crying. You can usually tell on the first night or two if it has any chance of success. On the first night your child may cry for half an hour before he settles down. On the next, if all goes well, the time will be shorter—say down to 20 minutes. Within a week the child will have learned that such crying is futile, and the problem will have been solved.

One mother wrote to me avidly praising the method. Her doctor had given her baby medicine to help him sleep, but the baby had broken out in a rash. To quote from her letter, "When the doctor saw the rash he put his prescription pad away and said 'let him cry.' I was anxious but pleased. If only he'd said that in the first place. All I needed was moral support, professional endorsement. That firm approach to 'let him cry' has given me more confidence in dealing with my children."

For this mother, and for many others, the method is undoubtedly a success. This particular mother knew what she wanted to do, but did not trust her own judgment. One of the most essential factors in dealing with sleep problems is to do what YOU believe is right. Do not worry about what experts, neighbors and relatives say if you feel happy in what you are doing and if it works. If you want to try the crying out approach and have been waiting for someone to tell you it is all right to do so, then go ahead.

There are, however, a great many parents for whom "crying out" seems totally unacceptable. There are many who have tried it and have run into problems. Unfortunately, far too many advisers in the past have implied that crying out is the only solution and that a parent who fails is not trying hard enough. This is far from the truth. There may be a large number of reasons why the method may fail. For a start, it may prove to be extremely impractical when the family lives in a small apartment or in a thin-walled house with nearby neighbors; and even more to the point, it goes against the parents' instincts. Nature has designed the cry to trigger off tremendously powerful emotions in parents. If the cry had not developed to have this effect it would have been useless to the child. In much the same way, the ringing of a telephone may be an intensely annoying noise, but it has been deliberately designed to be that way. If the sound were soothing, it could be ignored and would be valueless. The same goes for the cry.

When a mother hears a baby cry she knows that it is in distress, and to ignore the cry can be intolerably difficult. Indeed, at least one doctor has expressed concern that to do so deliberately may train a parent to be insensitive, rather than sensitive, to her children's needs.[1] It would seem that the "crying out" method has the best chance of success in cases where the parents themselves have conditioned the sleep problem. As an example, it may work well when a child has developed sleeplessness after being repeatedly brought downstairs during the evening to be shown to the parents' friends.

Most parents do try the "crying out" method. Like other doctors, I tend only to hear about the children for whom it has failed. If it has succeeded, then there is no problem and I don't hear about it again. In the letters I received from parents with long-term problems, a very large proportion expressed extreme disquiet and dissatisfaction with the method. As one mother wrote, "My doctor told me to let him scream. That has to be the most futile advice anyone can offer. A healthy child can scream for far longer than a shattered parent can stand." However, this advice is probably the most common given by doctors and other parents. Another mother quoted her doctor as saying, "You must be strong. Refuse to go and cuddle her for two weeks. You'll go through hell, but it will work." On the first night her child screamed for three hours. On the second she decided to give in and go to the child after listening to the scream from 2 A.M. until 4 A.M. I, for one, cannot blame her. An almost universal comment seemed to be, "I feel sure that the people who give this sort of advice have never had to face the problem themselves."

For the child who goes on screaming and screaming, the method still need not be a complete failure, but it does need to be better and more clearly organized. (See Chapter 11, "Behavior Therapy.") Other parents try different approaches. Some try to deal with the child who will not go to bed and stay there peacefully by getting him to go to sleep in the living room and then tiptoeing up to the bedroom with him in their arms, only to find him waking up the instant they lay him in his bed. Other parents try rides in the car, which often gets babies to sleep, but again the attempt to transfer the child to his room often fails.

The child who only settles for one parent and not the other at bedtime is being more deliberately manipulative and can cause tremendous resentment and worry for the parents. The parent who is allowed the honor of dealing with bedtime feels both secretly flattered and simultaneously annoyed at always being burdened with the task. The parent whose efforts are refused may feel rejected and angry, and possibly jealous.

More frequently than with other sleep difficulties, this particular problem can often be analyzed and traced back to its cause. In a majority of households the father does not return from work until shortly before the young child's bedtime. The two have not seen each other all day, and it is not surprising that they want to play together. Such games may become quite boisterous and it may happen that, as the two of them are dancing around together and enjoying a playful wrestle, mother comes in and announces that it is bedtime. Both father and child are put in their place like naughty schoolchildren, and it comes as no surprise that on being put to bed the child demands the father, refusing to cooperate with the mother. In this situation a further cause of problems is the child being put to bed straight after a playing session without a quiet time to wind down after all the fun and games.

At this point tremendous conflicts can arise. The mother may resent the fact that she spends all day looking after the child, cooking food, changing diapers, etc., while her husband is out of the house. It may seem unfair that he can appear to have the fun of having the child and not the work. This resentment can affect the mood of the house at bedtime. Alternatively, the father may feel that he is missing out on many shared experiences with the child and may feel deeply rejected if the child wants his mother to take him to bed.

Children are observant creatures and can quickly spot the effects that their behavior has on their parents. They may realize that one parent will be particularly kind or playful when he or she is selected and that the other is clearly upset when this happens. A child may even want to punish a parent who has told him off during the evening by rejecting him or her at bedtime.

If you are having problems like this yourselves, try to analyze what is happening in the family. Look at each person in turn and establish what effect this problem is having on him. If the child only allows one of you to take him to bed, try to find out why that one has been accepted and the other rejected. It may then be possible to alter your bedtime routine to deal with this.

One couple told me that they had particular success with this approach. Their daughter always insisted on going up to bed with Richard, her father. Richard would cuddle with her and read a story, and then sometimes he would put her to bed, and on other occasions Sally, his wife, would come in and try to take her. Sally was always rejected. The little girl would never settle down satisfactorily for her. Once they had analyzed what was going on in the household at bedtime the answer became obvious. Richard made certain that Sally was not always the one who was stuck in the kitchen while the pre-bedtime routine was underway. He would take an equal share in the preparation of the evening meal. Sally would have an equal number of evenings putting their daughter to bed. Richard had initially rejected the idea, saying that it was unfair that his wife could play with the child all day while the evening was his only opportunity. It took only a few days for them all to see what effect this attitude had been having, and to put it right.

THE BEDTIME ROUTINE

If bedtime were just a simple matter of taking a child up to his bed and saying good night, then it would still have enough potential problems to drive a parent to despair. It is not that simple. In fact, considering that the parent is attempting to turn a boisterous and mischievous bundle of energy into a calm and relaxed little angel, it is a miracle that children ever get to bed at all. Bedtime is, however, much more than going to bed. It is an elaborate ritual, often involving more emotional contact, more family traditions, and more pleasure than almost any other aspect of parenthood. Unfortunately and inevitably, any activity that can cause intense pleasure can also cause immense problems.

Modern life is lived in routines. Activity in a household tends to revolve around mealtimes, which in turn are affected by the time the adults and children have to go to work or school. Even a very young child will recognize, and get used to, the predictability of the pattern. There will be noise in the morning as people get dressed, varying degrees of chaos at breakfast, and then a peaceful lull when one of the parents and the older children have left the house. Such a pattern continues throughout the day and will be reassuring and settling to the young child.

When it comes to bedtime children certainly respond best to a continuation of the routine. In fact, of all the day's activities this is the one where a set routine is most advantageous. It doesn't matter if the actual time of going to bed varies or not, so long as the general routine is kept to. For children for whom bed has become something unpleasant, a place of tears of misery, the development of a happy routine can lower the emotional temperature considerably.

I certainly do not want to lay down rules as to when a child should go to bed. This is something that every family has to decide for itself. It is fair to say that some children are obviously put to bed too late, and others too early, but such comments can only be made after observing the effect on the child in question. What is "too late" for one child might be the "right" time for another. Perhaps the chief determinant of the best time for any given child is that child's own personality, and factors such as the time the child woke up in the morning and the amount of daytime sleep the child had are also very important. Certainly from my own experience, and that of almost every one of my correspondents, it is futile trying to buy an earlier or easier bedtime by keeping a child awake in the day. If a child is deliberately stopped from sleeping he will become overtired and irritable, both of which seem to lessen the chance of his going to sleep easily. By a cruel trick of nature, if a child does get even a short afternoon nap then the energy and wakefulness gained may keep him awake for an extra two to three hours.

It is clearly futile trying to put young children, particularly the two- to three-year olds, to bed if they are wide awake. Commonsense will tell you that you are simply wasting your time. Commonsense also says, quite correctly, that exercise before bedtime—particularly a vigorous game outside—will help a child settle down more easily. This obviously depends on an adequate routine being used in the transition between play and bed. To call a child in from playing outside and then send him straight to bed is clearly going to leave him keyed up and resentful, not to mention dirty. Even if he has only been playing with toys the process shouldn't be rushed. If you snatch the toys from him you are hardly likely to leave him relaxed. There is a danger of doing this when you have to go out yourselves—the very occasion when you least want him to act up for the babysitter. Plan ahead and take your time.

The actual time at which parents send their children to bed was looked at by the Newsons in their study of the care of urban four-year-olds.[2] They found that nearly 70% of the children went to bed between 6:30 and 8:00 P.M. In general, middle class parents sent their children to bed earlier than working class parents. In other societies the time will be quite different. Southern European children tend to go to bed much later, for example. However, the old concept that I certainly recall from my own childhood, that children of a certain age *must* be in bed by a set time, is no longer believed. It might nevertheless be a reasonable idea to stagger bedtimes slightly. The older child in a family can feel resentful if sent to bed at the same time as his younger brother or sister, and to keep him up a short while longer can be seen as both a privilege and his own "special" time to be alone with his parents.

One of the advantages in developing a particular routine at bedtime is that the child knows what is expected of him. If one night he is taken to bed and left alone, another night he has a story, and another night watches television, then he may become confused. Every family develops its own bedtime ritual, a ritual that often owes a lot to the parents' memory of their own childhood. I have heard of countless variations. One that has stood the test of time is the warm bath. Baths are an excellent way of preparing the child for bed. Not only will they, with any luck, get the child clean, but they are also relaxing and provide a natural interlude between play and bed. Baths should be fun, with sufficient time allowed for undressing and play, and they are obviously a private and intimate part of family life. Only the closest of friends or relatives who happen to be in the house at children's bedtime are usually allowed to watch or help. It is best to avoid battles at getting out time, though occasionally this is inevitable. Some children would gladly spend all night in a bath, provided they were allowed to keep filling it up with hot water. The cuddling that follows the bath also gives an otherwise independent child a chance to be babied, to regress to the physical contact that they so often reject at other times.

After a child is dried and dressed in his pajamas, there is often a short period before it is actually time to go to bed. This is clearly not a time for exciting games, but a time for cuddling, for relaxing, for being together as a family. I may sound dreadfully reactionary for saying it, but I do feel that television has here diminished the pleasure of family life. Watching television has in many families supplanted the bedtime story, the nursery rhymes, and the lullabies. Perhaps similar complaints were made by storytellers when printing was invented, but there seems to be far more intimacy and enjoyment in sharing a story than in sharing a ready-made slice of someone else's entertainment. I do not believe television is in any way harmful, but is is sad if there is more communication between the broadcasters and the children than between the parents and their children. There are many households where this is the case.

I am probably here not only hankering back to bedtime as it was when I was a child but am also following the class difference in attitudes towards stories. The Newsons, in their study, found massive differences between different social groups. For example, while a majority of middle class parents read their children a story, only one in seven parents did this where the breadwinner was an unskilled worker. The Newsons commented that the working class parents tended to see stories as a childish indulgence, whereas the middle class parents saw them as far more important—both socially and educationally.

It is never too early to start to read to a child. Don't wait until he is old enough to understand stories, songs, or nursery rhymes. Rhymes in particular have a rhythm that even the youngest child can enjoy, and for a baby to sit on a parent's knee as he or she looks through and talks about a picture book is far from a waste of time. In fact, activities like this, even in the youngest child, help begin to prepare him or her for reading. Such skills as appreciating which way the eyes move across the page, and the fact that books are fun, can help the child to associate reading with pleasure rather than with work. Similarly, there is no need to stop reading when a child is old enough to read stories to himself. I know of many families where the teenagers still have, and enjoy, a bedtime story, though they would be mortified if their friends found out.

Many children enjoy hearing the same story over and over again. Christopher must have asked me to read one particular little book hundreds of times. This seemingly silly story of a tiger who eats all the food and drink in a bemused family's house seemed to hold intense fascination for him. I got bored. If, after the first fifty or so readings, I changed a word to try and shorten it, he would complain. Children may know a story by heart, but can still derive pleasure and security from hearing it yet again.

Perhaps the most successful writer of children's books in the world is Roald Dahl. His stories, such as *Charlie & the Chocolate Factory, The Twits,* and *James and the Giant Peach,* have delighted countless children at bedtime and have sufficient humor and story line to keep long-suffering parents happy while they read them aloud. As I read them to my children I was often struck by the fact that chapters frequently ended on a frightening note, and yet the children went to sleep quite happily. Roald Dahl explained that he tried to write chapters of a specific length to be read in bed and often finished them on an exciting note. "I don't believe that any children are given nightmares or any other kind of fears by the things I write. Whenever I write anything 'nasty' it is always tempered by humor so that the laugh dissipates fear in the listener. In my opinion the sort of thing that would give the child nightmares would be sheer humorless bloodthirstiness or humorless horror in stories, and I never do that. The secret surely lies in getting it to be funny all the time and mixing the funniness with a swiftly moving plot, and plenty of tension.''

Another immensely successful children's writer, says that he feels that younger children need books with a picture on each page and a joke at the end, and that parents need material that they can read in five minutes so that the bedtime story does not end up too long. Thank heavens that some writers know what parents need, but then they do know who chooses the books!

Stories can also be made up by the parents, and many successful children's writers started by inventing stories for their own children. But whether read or made up, stories provide a close verbal communication between parent and child. Such verbal communication can also come from sitting on the child's bed and having a little private chat about the day's events, or the day to come. Such discussions are often trivial, but can be immensely beneficial to both parent and child. Depending on one's religious views, prayers together have much the same function.

The other commonly used verbal method is the singing of nursery rhymes or lullabies. Nursery rhymes get handed down from generation to generation, although their place in a children's repertoire is now being invaded by television advertising jingles. The short, tuneful, catchiness of such jingles is what attracts youngsters, whether or not they have the slightest idea what the words are about. Lullabies are often traditional too, but many parents make up their own. The occasional lullaby even makes its way into songwriters' repertoires. Tom Paxton, for one, has recorded several beautiful lullabies that he wrote for his own children, *Jennifer's Rabbit* being perhaps the best known. Other examples include Paul Simon's *St. Judy's Comet,* which exudes a desperation at not being able to get his son to sleep that we have all felt, and John Lennon's moving lullaby to his son Sean, *Beautiful Boy*.

Many children have a warm drink while listening to a story or watching television. This helps the child to wind down, but there is considerable evidence that such drinks can actually improve the quality of sleep. No research has, to my knowledge, been carried out recently with children, but several studies have looked at the effects on adults.

Milk contains an amino acid called L-Tryptophan which may well have sleep-inducing properties itself. Some adult insomniacs now take tablets of this safe chemical, and in their book *Natural Sleep,* Philip Goldberg and Daniel Kaufman discuss and enthuse about the possibilities of this chemical at length.[6] They do not consider the effects of L-Tryptophan on children. But if the current theories are correct this may go some way towards explaining the soporific effects of milk drinks at bedtime. Incidentally, the Newsons found that 43% of infants were given a bottle or pacifier to take to bed with them, and in addition, a third of them were given a warm drink before being put to bed. At the time of the survey this was against standard advice and many parents felt very guilt about it.

Because young babies often settle down after a feeding, many parents go on to give them a pacifier even after they have finished bottle or breast feeding. Provided that they are clean and not dipped in or contain any sweet substances that could harm the teeth, pacifiers are harmless. Parents often worry that their children will not grow out of them, but how many adults did you see today with a pacifier? Cigarettes or pipes as a substitute, maybe, but pacifiers never. Some parents worry about hygiene and boil the pacifier. This is only logical if thumb suckers have their thumbs boiled, too, which is clearly impractical. Both need washing, certainly, but there is no need to be obsessive.

While some children suck their thumbs and others choose a pacifier, many more settle into bed with an old teddy bear, piece of rag, or other scruffy object that they like to cuddle. Called "transitional objects" by psychologists, they are often used after the mother has left the child at night and somehow seem to be a form of substitute mother. I have heard such pieces of rag or blanket called a "snuckler," "cuddly," "doo-doo," "snuggly," "ayah," "foofer," "thumbrag," "fluff," "sleepy," and "beddy." They are often bizarre, and parents may not be able to explain why a child became attached to one particular object. Christopher used a shabby old blanket and became desperately upset if it was taken from him, if only to be washed. (It did become revolting at times.) Once such blankets are washed they seem to lose their appeal temporarily. Even the smell seems to be important. Katy never used one. She put the thumb of one hand in her mouth, and with the other hand held on tightly to the hair at the crown of her head. It was her bedtime ritual, and who were we to complain?

There is no need to worry that the child will not give up the "cuddly" in time. He will. It may take a long time, but since it is harmless, stop worrying about it. As a last thought on the subject, it appears that in the non-literate societies where children share beds and therefore have far more tactile stimulation from their parents, transitional objects are virtually unknown.

Finally the child is left in his or her bed. Parents often leave with a few ritualized standard words such as, "Good night. God Bless. See you in the morning," and kiss the child good night. At least a third of parents have some specific ritual for these last few moments,[2] and sensible hospital authorities wisely allow parents to put their hospitalized children to bed and to follow their own ritual there. The security that the child feels from such familiarity can be very rewarding.

THE NEW BABY

The sleep problems of babies are discussed throughout the book, particularly in Chapter 4, "Simple Sleep Problems," and Chapter 10, "Bed-sharing." However, there are a few suggestions that are worth making here.

It is usual for babies in the first month or so to be wrapped securely when put to bed, but the position the child lies in does not really matter. Occasionally the very young become frustrated if left on their stomachs by being unable to turn over or see around, and such frustration may lead to crying. After the first few months it makes no difference where you put the child. He'll soon end up somewhere else!

There does not appear to be any real evidence that a baby is likely to choke if he is lying on his back and vomits. The dangers have probably been exaggerated as a normal baby will always move his head if his position prevents him from breathing. The risk seems the same whatever the position. It is, however, sensible to wrap a young baby firmly since a newborn baby left lying naked will flail about wildly. Gentle pressure on the abdomen will calm him rapidly, and wrapping him up firmly has the same soothing effect.

If all else has failed and you still have a crying baby who refuses to settle down, one interesting recent invention does seem to offer some relief. This is a simple rocking device which consists of a spring that can be attached to the ceiling or door frame and a nylon hammock in which you put the baby's basket. It rocks gently up and down at a constant 65 times a minute, propelled only by an occasional gentle push.

Research workers have investigated such devices at considerable length.[7] At a rocking rate of 30 times per minute crying continues. If the rate is gradually increased crying almost always stops within 15 seconds when a rate of 60-70 times per minute is reached. On stopping the rocking after a couple of minutes the babies usually remain quiet. The research on which the device is based is certainly impressive and it does seem to have helped many parents.

Rocking is not the only rhythmical sensation that can settle a baby down. Music and other background noise can have a very powerful hypnotic effect. A few years ago claims were made from Japan that recordings of the sounds a baby would hear while in the uterus were very soothing to the crying newborn baby. Such recordings are still available and their most impressive results are usually obtained with the very young child. In one report every one of 403 crying infants was calmed within 41 seconds of the record being started.[8] A later report showed equally impressive results and also showed that neither the maternal heartbeat nor a metronome soothed newborn infants. However, the intrauterine sounds lose their soothing properties within a few weeks of the infant's birth.

Perhaps the most bizarre method for helping a young child get to sleep is covered by U.S. Patent 3552388. This consists of a device which is supposed to work by means of periodic pats on the baby's bottom.[9] I don't think I can recommend it! Such gimmicks are nowhere near as important as adopting a happy and relaxed routine leading up to bedtime, and no one can ever patent that!

· 6 ·

Disturbed Nights

NIGHT WAKING

Night waking is by far the most common of all the problems that cause parents concern. The frustration and despair that it can cause is immense. One mother named Mary, wrote to me at length of her feelings, and it is worth quoting her in full. Her child was four and "she had, by this time, established a kind of pattern—waking up between twelve and two and staying awake for up to two hours, sometimes longer. Putting her to bed later had no significant effect. I couldn't follow the doctor's advice and let her cry because after a few minutes my husband would be driven to desperation. He had a responsible and very demanding job which required all his physical stamina. I must admit I rather resented the fact that it was always my job to go to her and keep her silent so that he could sleep. The trouble seemed to be that by 1 A.M. she needed a couple of hours of wakeful activity. I sang songs and read books and told stories night after night, often falling asleep in mid-sentence, whereupon little fingers would pry open my eyelids and she would prompt me with the next words of the story or song which she knew by heart."

Many parents tell the same story—and many mothers also express intense resentment at having to get up at night while their

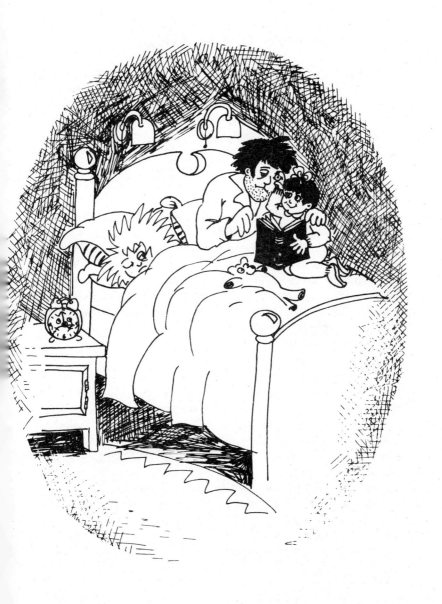

husbands sleep. I was troubled at the phrase in Mary's letter saying that she accepted that her husband needed to sleep because he had a "responsible and very demanding job." What is motherhood if not responsible and very demanding? I firmly believe that parents should share the responsibility, but I accept that many will disagree. One mother quoted her family doctor's comments when she had said that her husband helped her by getting up at night. The doctor was quite adamant. "You must never let him do that, dear," she was told. "Your husband has a job to go to. You've got nothing to do all day. You should get up." The intriguing thing about that quote was that the doctor was a woman.

In Chapters 3 and 4 I looked at many of the possible reasons for night waking, but—whatever the cause—parents try an incredible number of techniques to get some rest. A father told me of the things he and his wife had tried, and if the exhaustion did not come shining through, the list might almost sound amusing. He tried "leaving the light on, and turning it off, drinks, cookies, toys in her room, no toys in her room, a pillow, more blankets, less blankets, less noise downstairs, more noise downstairs, leaving a ticking clock in the bedroom, playing soft music on a tape, and," he added with more than a little feeling, "yelling at her." In the end, after talking to other suffering parents he decided that all these things were a waste of time and that it was simply a matter of surviving until she did start to sleep through the night, which eventually she did.

Another mother described her experience: "His cry on waking was terrible. This has been verified by experienced mothers who admitted that they had previously thought I had been exaggerating the problem and had been too soft and anxious. So how did we cope? We tried every remedy or course of action we heard of from friends, parents, books, the doctor, etc. I don't think we tried anything you won't hear from other people. The point is that nothing worked, but we coped by always having something else to try and keeping up this desperate optimism that the next thing we tried would be *IT*."

Parental management can sometimes aggravate the problem,

and the parent who is totally inconsistent in dealing with a wakeful child is almost certainly asking for trouble. To alternate from taking the child into your own bed one day, and then expecting it to cry itself back to sleep the next, must surely confuse the child. Nevertheless, the research quoted in Chapter 3 showed that most of the techniques employed by parents were simply a response to the problem and not the cause of it. I am certain that this is correct, but commonsense dictates that you should stick to one approach at a time.

You may decide that you want to sit with your child holding his hand until he goes back to sleep. If so, don't try it for just one night and then decide the next night that you are too tired and go in and shout at him. Similarly, if you believe that bedsharing is the answer, commit yourself to doing this regularly, not just on those nights when you cannot face sitting up with your child.

Put yourself in your child's position. Once awake, would you not become terribly confused if every night something different happened to you? If there were nights when you woke at 10:30 and your parents were still up and on some occasions happy to play with you, read a story, or enjoy cuddling? As a child, would you be able to understand it if you woke the next night at 3 A.M. and your parents reacted completely differently—if, instead of being happy to have you with them, they seemed angry and resentful? Would this not make you still more confused and anxious?

As one letter writer said, it can be helpful to keep trying different techniques until you find a way of coping. Nevertheless, you should try to adopt each for at least a week—not simply a night—before attempting something new. It is important to remember that there is one rule of sleep problems: one day the problem will disappear. One day either your children will sleep or else they will learn to entertain themselves when they wake without disturbing you. The problem is that I cannot tell you which day it will be! Mind you, it is always possible that it will be tomorrow, and I think the "desperate optimism" described by the letter writer I quoted earlier is very important. To keep yourself going, you do need either to remain optimistic, or else learn to accept the problem, getting your rest in whatever way you can, and without getting angry.

Extreme anger is a very common emotion when parents are woken at night. As another mother told me, "I would lie there absolutely rigid, refusing to go to him and praying that he would go back to sleep. Consequently I increased his fears and added to his insecurity." She went on, having analyzed her feelings at length, "My continual refusal to respond can only be interpreted as rejection, and distrust is planted. During the night in the dark and quiet this must be very frightening. Fear prevents relaxation, and the sleeplessness goes on."

Her conclusion, one shared by many advisers, is that if the mother can just relax, the child will sense this and will settle down to sleep better. However, please realize that while this is undoubtedly true, the opposite does not automatically apply. If a child does not settle down it does not necessarily mean that he is sensing his mother's tension.

Babies are particularly sensitive to their parents' emotions. If you are cuddling a baby who is crying, and you feel upset, your own arm muscles will be tense and rigid. There is no doubt that babies are aware of this. Often they settle down if passed to someone else for whom the crying is not such a source of worry. I have often seen parents cuddling a screaming baby in the hospital look on in amazement when he is taken by a nurse, for whom he promptly settles. Such parents may deny that they feel tense. However, feeling the arm muscles as they hold the child can reveal tremendous muscular tension. Try to let your muscles go loose. Deliberately let them go floppy. It is perfectly easy to hold the child gently with relaxed rather than tense arms. Try it. Both you and the child will sense the difference.

At a less subtle level, it is also perfectly obvious that a child will not find it easy to go back to sleep if you storm into its room, turn the light full on, and accuse it at the top of your voice of deliberately making your life miserable. This may be obvious, but almost everyone has done it.

While I have looked here at what the parents do when their child wakes at night, John and Elizabeth Newson have also looked at what the child does. Of the four-year-olds that they observed, 6% lay in bed talking or singing until they went back to sleep, 37% called out, 34% cried, 10% got out of bed to find their parents, 5% apparently never woke, and the remaining 8% resorted to numerous other tricks such as banging their heads against the pillow.[1] In other words, over eight out of ten adopted behavior that would end up in their parents being woken up.

The Newsons also asked the parents how they would cope with this waking spell. Almost all said they would go and reassure the child. And while 34% said that they would never allow the child into their bed, the others concluded that the greatest reassurance came from doing just that. This is such an important and controversial area that I devote a chapter to it (see Chapter 10, "Bed-sharing").

EARLY WAKING

Frustrating as it may be to be woken from your sleep by a child at an unusually early hour, such as five o'clock in the morning, it is relatively simple to deal with if it is an isolated problem. Unfortunately, it rarely is. The early waker may also have woken up several times during the night, or have caused you problems at bedtime. If this is the case, then the problems and possible solutions are discussed elsewhere.

If early waking is an isolated problem, then by far the simplest answer is to adjust your life style and your own sleeping times to fit your child's. It is much easier to go to bed at nine o'clock and get up at five than it is to go to bed at midnight and persuade your child to stay asleep until seven. Believe me, I've tried both ways. There is a bonus, too. Early morning can be the most pleasant time of day, with clean crisp sunshine that has disappeared by the time that most people have their breakfast.

If you are not feeling quite so philosophical about early waking, and in particular if your social life or working hours control your sleeping habits, then it is worth trying to find out if there is any one thing that wakes your child. There may be a train passing on a nearby track at the same early hour each day; birds may be nesting near your child's bedroom window and waking him with their dawn singing; or an increasing amount of traffic may be building up on the road outside. Occasionally, the noise of a time-controlled central heating system starting up may wake a child who is only at a shallow level of sleep. It may even be the lightness of the room. Some children seem to stay asleep longer in the dark, and while thin curtains keep the room dark during the night, they may not keep out bright sunlight. Thicker or darker curtains may be the answer here.

When your child is old enough, make sure that he has something to occupy him when he wakes so that he need not wake you. This may mean having some sort of light switch, often a string from the ceiling within his reach. Provide books, toys, and a drink. Make it clear to him that he must stay in his room, and keep your fingers firmly crossed. The older the child, the more likely it is that this approach will succeed. When it does work it is a total success for everyone concerned, but there can sometimes be snags. When we tried it with Christopher he would still come into our room at 5:30 in the morning, asking for help with the model spaceship he had tried to build. The adult concept of time was still beyond him. Sometimes you just can't win.

You will have noticed that I have not made any attempt to define early waking. This is because the description "early" is relative to the time the parents wake up. If you are a farmer who always gets up at five o'clock and your child sleeps until 5:30, then he is certainly not "early" in the context of your family. If you do not normally get up until eight, then 5:30 may seem unacceptably early. Certainly I would not consider that a child who sleeps until half an hour before the time you wake to have a sleeping problem. Despite this, I have known parents who sometimes ask for medicine to make their child sleep this extra thirty minutes.

• 7 •

Restless Sleep

Even when children do get off to sleep satisfactorily, all manner of new problems may arise during the night. The ideal is for everyone to drift happily off to sleep, blissfully slumber the hours of darkness away, and wake the next morning happy and refreshed.

It's lovely when it happens, but this picture of domestic bliss may be interrupted by a variety of relatively minor, but nonetheless irritating problems. Every child dreams, but many have nightmares that leave them awake and terrified. Other children may talk or walk in their sleep, grind their teeth, bang their heads on the pillow, or wet their beds. One of the most common night disturbances in the younger child is the night terror, in which he or she is found screaming, but not fully awake. Such children may take a long time to calm down, and yet in the morning be oblivious of their adventures in the night.

It is always difficult to estimate exactly how common such disturbances are. Quite a lot is known about their relative incidence, however. One researcher showed that over all age groups sleepwalking is only half as common as night terrors, which are only a quarter as common as nightmares.[1] When he analyzed the types of disturbance experienced by children at different ages he found remarkable differences. For example, in the group of

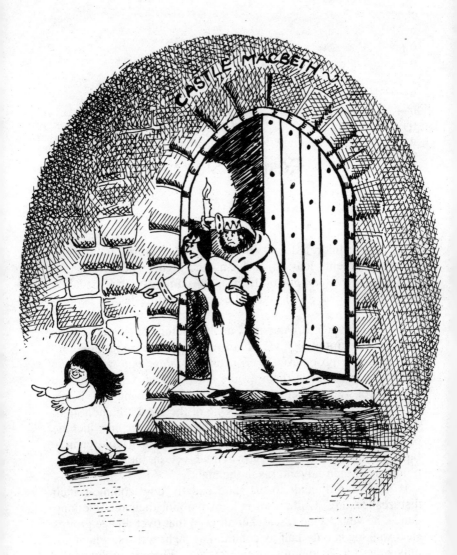

"Look, I told you it was hereditary."

children with sleep disturbances that he looked at, he found that night terrors were experienced by 63% of the four- to seven-year-olds, 24% of the eight- to ten-year-olds, and had gone down to only 13% in the eleven- to fourteen-year-old age group.

Nightmares were rather different. For example, while they were a problem for only 19% of the four- to seven-year-olds, they had shot up to as many as 69% in the eight to ten age group, and then had dropped to 12% of the eleven- to 14-year-olds. In other words, there was a dramatic peak in the incidence of nightmares between eight and ten.

Only 5% of four- to seven-year-olds with sleep disturbances were sleepwalking, going up steadily to 30% at eight to ten and after this age it was the major problem, being the complaint in 65% of the children.

It can be seen that each of these problems has a completely different age pattern, and in addition the sex ratio altered substantially as well. At age four to seven years, boys were twice as likely as girls to have these problems, but by eleven to fourteen they were twenty times more likely to have them. Quite a difference.

For many years doctors and parents thought that most of these experiences were associated with dreaming. It seemed likely that the child who woke up screaming in terror must be dreaming, or that sleepwalkers and talkers were somehow acting out their dreams. Even bed-wetting was, and often still is, assumed to have a connection with dreaming.

Such ideas have been radically changed by the arrival of the electroencephalogram. EEG recordings have shown clearly that dreams and nightmares are associated with Rapid Eye Movement sleep but that the other problems are not. Bed-wetting, sleepwalking, sleep talking and night terrors are all associated with emergence from stage 3 and stage 4 non-REM sleep. As a result they have been termed "disorders of arousal."

These various disorders often appear in the same person at different times, and there is often a family history of such problems.[2] Indeed, as well as being associated with the same stage of sleep, they have several other features in common. They all occur in paroxysms—for example, one week in three—and they are characterized by a lack of response to the child's surroundings, and are forgotten on waking.

There is other evidence that these disturbances are not merely an extension of dreaming. All these upsets occur chiefly in the first three hours of sleep, whereas REM sleep occurs mainly in the last third of the night. EEG studies have also shown that the upsets occur in REM sleep in less than 10% of recordings. In addition, waking from REM sleep nearly always results in a dream being remembered, but the child who is woken when bed-wetting or sleepwalking remembers nothing.

Despite their similarities, these different night disturbances are worth considering individually. The particular problem of bed-wetting, which causes distress to tens of thousands of parents and children, has a chapter to itself.

DREAMS AND NIGHTMARES

Dreams have always fascinated man. They seem so real, and yet are intangible. No one can be sure where they come from or why they happen, even though plenty of people have offered suggestions. Indeed, attempts to interpret the meaning of dreams date back to the Old Testament.

Over the years attitudes to dreams have varied enormously. In Ancient Egypt dreams were thought to be a form of communication from the supernatural, and officially approved dreaming areas were set up where it was thought that such dreams were more likely to happen. By the Middle Ages dreams were usually seen as warnings of unpleasant events to come, and this mystical view of dreams as somehow coming from outside the person continued up to the late 17th century. From then on it was realized that dreaming was simply a function of the mind, as expressed by Daniel Defoe who wrote, "To dream is nothing else but to think sleeping."

From this change of attitude it was only a short step to the analysis of dreams as a means of understanding the dreamer. Sigmund Freud wrote and studied this aspect of dreaming at great length, and in 1899 published his book *The Interpretation of Dreams*. From that time his name has been a household word.

The psychiatrists and psychoanalysts who followed Freud all produced their own ideas and theories. To me the interpretations suggested by Freud, Jung, Adler, Hall, Gutheil, and many others, tell us a lot more about them and their fantasies than it does about the dreamer. On a less serious level, many books have been published listing the possible meanings of symbols and events in dreams. If you were hoping that one of these would help you analyze your child's nighttime adventures, then I'm afraid you will be disappointed. Such generalizations are quite fun on the level of a party game, but are meaningless as a serious scientific or medical tool. Dream symbols cannot simply be translated like a foreign language.

The EEG has fundamentally changed our views of dreams. Freud thought that one of the functions of dreams was to preserve sleep, but it now seems that one of the functions of sleep is to allow dreaming. As I mentioned in Chapter 2, depriving someone of their REM sleep can be damaging.

A majority of dreams are either pleasant or simply boring, and they may become a problem for young children when they become frightening. In 1920 a Dr. Kimmins did some fascinating research, collecting the dreams of thousands of children.[3] He found that a fourth of all the dreams reported were frightening, and in a majority of these the frightening image was that of an old man. He also found that children up to the age of six or seven often confused dreaming and waking. For example, they might dream they were given a toy, and would search their room for it on waking up.

It is difficult to know why children have frightening dreams and nightmares. Hugh Jolly feels that children who have them are generally brighter than average and advises that such children may need to avoid excessive excitement just before bedtime. Other pediatricians have suggested that colds or nasal obstructions may trigger nightmares, particularly ones about suffocation and drowning.

There is no doubt that nightmares are more common when the

child is anxious or worried. If they are happening very frequently, say every night, then they are likely to be due to insecurity such as some unhappiness at school or at home.[4] It is rarely useful to ask a child what he is worried about. It makes far more sense just to keep an eye on him, watching his games and drawings, as very often the cause of his worry will make itself apparent. You can certainly talk about the problem once you have found out what it is, and this alone may help to end the nightmares. Obviously, if the nightmare keeps happening and you cannot sort it out yourself, then it is worth asking your doctor's advice.

Martin Herbert, the prominent psychologist, has commented that nightmares are particularly noticeable in children who have a period of separation from their mothers, especially if this runs to a period of four weeks or longer.[5] This is even more likely if the child is in a hospital. If separated from his mother, but still sleeping in his own home, the child is less likely to have the problem.

One factor that has often been blamed for nigthmares is television. It has been said that a frightening program at bedtime is more likely to lead to a disturbed night. In 1964 an investigation was carried out with two groups of volunteer children. Each group was shown a TV program. One group saw a bloody western and the other a romantic comedy, but to the disappointment of the scientists neither group dreamed of the show they had seen. However, the group that saw the western certainly had more vivid, even if not particularly frightening, dreams. It would seem to be common sense to advise that children should not watch very exciting or frightening programs immediately before they go to bed. This is not really because of the risk of nightmares, but because they are likely to find it harder to get to sleep.

Many people do believe that the influences of television on their children can be harmful. One mother wrote to me about her seven-year-old daughter who dreamt almost every night of ghosts. It is worth quoting her letter directly. "I told my doctor who recommended censoring her TV and reading material. Fine, but you cannot censor children's talk and she would talk to her friends about ghosts, and look at books about them at school. The doctor also suggested leaving a light on (she had three), leaving the door open (we always have)." The poor doctor could not win, and eventually a hypnotherapist was approached who did help—probably by teaching an improved technique of bedtime relaxation.

As a final point in this brief review of dreams and nightmares, there is little doubt that children who share their bed or bedroom have fewer unpleasant dreams. Many families who have reared their children both in their own separate rooms and in a communal family bed have said that sleeping together leads to a reduction of unpleasant dreams almost immediately.

Causes aside, if your child is having a nightmare, what should you do?

For a start you should get to him as quickly as possible and sit and comfort him. Try to take his mind off the nightmare. There is no point in talking about its content then. Leave that until the morning. Instead, try talking about something calm and pleasant. Comfort and reassurance from the parent is a wonderful cure.

NIGHT TERRORS

Many parents confuse night terrors with nightmares, but they are very different. A child with a night terror will be found screaming, sitting up, wide-eyed, with dilated pupils, and very frightened and agitated. He doesn't recognize his parents during the attack and is disoriented. Comforting hardly seems to help. The child may sometimes thrash around, have a very rapid pulse, breathe fast, and sweat profusely.

These upsetting episodes last an average of two mintues, though they may last anywhere from one to twenty minutes. The only thing a parent can do is hold the child until he settles down and goes back to sleep. Thankfully, the entire episode will not be recalled.

There is little doubt that night terrors and sleepwalking have many links. They both occur at the same stage of sleep and both run in families. A study of twins has shown that if one twin suffers from either of these problems then the other twin is six times as likely to suffer as well if they are identical twins, rather than non-identical. This finding definitely suggests a genetic rather than environmental cause.[6] Similarly, in 80% of sleepwalkers, and 96% of those suffering from night terrors, a close relative was known to have had one or both conditions.[7]

Stress can make attacks more frequent, but is rarely the cause. The night terrors will eventually stop. They are harmless, however distressing they may appear at the time, and they leave no long- or short-term effects other than a disturbed night for the family.

If no particular stress can be uncovered and dealt with, and the episodes are becoming very frequent, then the benzodiazepine drugs such as Diazepam (Valium), or Flurazepam (Dalmane) have been shown to help. As with all drugs in childhood, these should only be used when they are really necessary.

SLEEPWALKING

It has been estimated that around 15% of children have sleep-walked at least once, although it is rare before five years old. The majority of somnambulists are between ten and fourteen and eventually outgrow the condition, although it still occasionally affects around 2% of adults.[8]

It is a curious condition. The sleepwalker's eyes may be open, but he cannot really see. He can navigate his way around a house, and yet lacks any real critical judgment of what he is doing. It is certainly possible for a sleepwalker to fall downstairs or through a window. The walker is asleep, but not dreaming, and the EEG shows the walking to occur at the transition from stages 3 and 4 non-REM sleep to the lighter stages. One researcher found that sleepwalking could be induced in 7 of 38 sleepwalkers by standing them up during stage 3 or 4 non-REM sleep, but could not be induced in REM sleep. Normal controls could not be made to walk at any stage.

The sleep EEG of somnambulists has shown the presence of sudden bursts of slow frequency waves before walking. These bursts are present in some 85% of normal six- to eleven-month-old babies, but are only present in 3% of seven- to nine-year-olds. This might well be due to a mild degree of central nervous system immaturity, and the eventual disappearance of the behavior in most adults represents maturation.

A typical sleepwalking episode consists of the child suddenly sitting bolt upright in bed, eyes open but unseeing. He gets up, may open cupboards or doors as if looking for something, and moves with somewhat clumsy movements. It is usually fruitless trying to talk to the sleepwalker, as questions may be answered with a grunt or have no bearing on the question. The episode ends with the child making his way back to bed and going back to sleep. In true somnambulism nothing of what happened will be remembered the next day.

I have already discussed the genetic aspects of sleepwalking when dealing with night terrors, and again it must be stressed that sleepwalking in itself does not mean that a child has emotional problems. As a leading medical journal article pointed out, the best known fictional example of sleepwalking must surely be Lady Macbeth, "whose nocturnal obsessional handwashing was closely related to the life stresses that she brought on herself by her ambitious personality."[9] Such images have made many people associate somnambulism with stress, and indeed, 81% of adult sleepwalkers feel that they are more likely to sleepwalk if under pressure. With children this seems to be less often the case, although those who are genetically predisposed to sleepwalking may be more likely to do so just before exams or during other periods of stress.

What can you do about it? It certainly helps to establish a relaxed and happy bedtime routine, particularly for those children in whom stress is a major factor. Many myths exist about sleepwalking, one of which is that somnambulists never injure themselves. Sadly this is not true. As many as 24% of adult sleepwalkers have reported injuring themselves, and injuries to children have certainly been reported. It makes good sense to apply some basic protective measures, such as locking large bedroom windows or blocking off the stairs.

Any number of treatments have been tried for persistent sleepwalking and it is worth consulting your doctor if it keeps happening, although occasional episodes are of no concern. Treatments have included drugs, adjusting the sleeping arrangements in the house, and psychotherapy. The most effective drugs, as with night terrors, are the benzodiazepine drugs which act by reducing the amount of stage 4 non-REM sleep and by reducing the number of shifts from one stage of sleep to another. Long-term use is, of course, best avoided. But for the short-term they can be extremely effective.

Two rather unconventional methods have also come to my notice. The first, thankfully, failed. The parent had tied the sleepwalking child into bed in a desperate attempt to stop him from walking. On the first night, while fast asleep, he untied the knots and went for his walk as usual. The second method had far more to commend it. After every other method had failed, the child's grandmother secretly knitted a small embroidered blanket. She gave it to the child and told her it was a "magic" blanket sent by the fairies to stop her walking at night. Afterward, the child slept with her head on it and never sleepwalked again!

SLEEP TALKING

The medical name for sleepwalking has a pleasant ring to it; "somnambulism" somehow sounds right. But the name for sleep talking is unlikely ever to become common usage. Somniloquy is rarely a major problem for children, unless they talk so loudly that they disturb the household. For adults it can be much more of a hazard, depending on who they are talking about and who they are sleeping with!

Sleep talking in children is frequently associated with episodes of somnambulism, but when it occurs alone it is again usually associated with non-REM sleep, and therefore not with dreaming. The talk itself is usually incomprehensible, and it is pointless trying to enter a conversation with a sleep talking child. Sleep talking certainly does not mean your child has psychiatric problems. There is no need to treat sleep talking if it is an isolated problem, and a child will not wake himself up simply by talking in his sleep.

TEETH GRINDING AND EXCESSIVE MOVEMENTS

Teeth grinding, or bruxism, can occur both in the daytime and during sleep. It involves the forced contraction of the muscles used in chewing and results in the intensely irritating noise of the teeth being ground together. It occurs chiefly in stage 1 or 2 sleep, and may be preceded by an increase in the heart rate and other body movements. It can certainly be severe enough to cause significant damage to the teeth and gums. Whether it is caused by poor occlusion of the teeth or emotional stress, it is difficult to be certain. Treatment can involve the benzodiazepine drugs, rubber tooth guards, relaxation techniques, or even hypnosis. If it is only mild it is not worth treating.

There are other involuntary movements that can occur during sleep and cause concern to parents. Head banging, or to give it its rather splendid medical name, Jactation Capitis Nocturna, consists of a violent rhythmic hitting of the head against a pillow, or sometimes rocking the body while going to sleep. These movements occur just before falling asleep, or during sleep. It usually starts in infancy and rapidly fades away; it occasionally persists, particularly, but not always, in children of below-average intelligence. It is harmless and leaves no ill effects, and the only management required is to ensure that whatever the child hits his head on is at least soft.

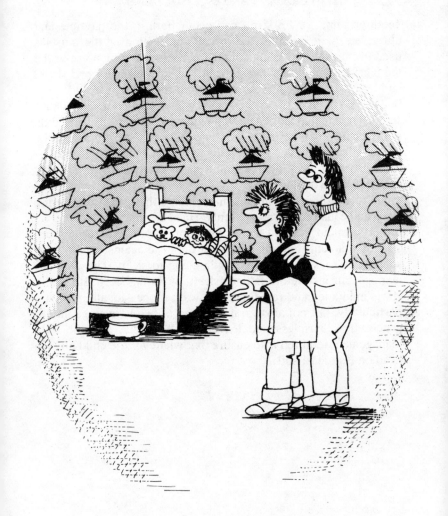

"Perhaps if we changed the wallpaper?"

• 8 •

Bed-wetting

Bed-wetting probably causes more concern than all the other problems that can occur during sleep. Otherwise known as nocturnal enuresis, it can turn bedtime from being the relaxed enjoyable time that we would all like it to be into a stressful time of anxiety and argument. The child whose every trip to bed ends in his feeling embarrassed and upset is hardly likely to look forward to bedtime with eager anticipation.

Bed-wetting only becomes a problem when a child continues to wet at night after the majority of children have become dry. There is no sudden dividing line between the normal and the abnormal. The natural history of acquiring bladder control is summarized below, but do remember my warnings, about such "average" descriptions, in Chapter 2. The child who does not fit this schedule exactly is not necessarily "abnormal."

The very young infant has virtually no bladder control. The bladder gradually fills, and when it is sufficiently distended, it empties. Indeed, it is rare for the child to have any significant bladder control before he can walk. After all, if you can't get to the potty, there is no point in waiting. Around fifteen to eighteen months the child usually becomes able to tell his mother that he has wet his diaper, and shortly afterward says that he wants to go, but doesn't give her time to do anything about it. By eighteen to twenty-four months he is able to tell his mother in time to be brought to the potty or bathroom, and by two to tow-and-a-half years he can go by himself. The three-year-old may be able to get through the night dry if he is taken to the potty at his parents' bedtime.

Approximately nine out of ten children become dry at night sometime between one-and-a-half and four-and-a-half years, usually sometime during the third year. In common with other skills like walking and talking, there is considerable variation. Control of bowel function usually comes before control of the bladder, but even after becoming dry all children can temporarily become wet if they are upset.

In their impressive study of seven hundred four-year-olds,[1] John and Elizabeth Newson found that at that particular age 27% of children sometimes wet their bed, 19% wet their bed once a week or more, and 11% had more wet nights than dry ones. The bed-wetting caused considerable problems for the families concerned. Indeed, very few mothers of enuretic children were not bothered by it. The ones who were least concerned were those who had an older child who had also been enuretic and had learned not only how to cope with it but also that the problem eventually ceases.

The reasons to get upset are numerous. As the Newsons pointed out, shortly after a baby is born the appearance of diapers on a wash line displays to the world that the happy event has occurred. It is even something to be proud of. If diapers are still hanging out four years later, many parents feel that they have somehow failed.

There are other practical problems. The child who is deep asleep tends to empty his bladder completely, leaving a bed that is not merely damp, but soaking. The problems of laundry, of smells, and of the general management of the mess can often make a mother despair if she is simply told by her doctor or friends that her child will grow out of it.

Before considering what can be done about bed-wetting, it is worth quickly examining the theories as to why it happens. In an attempt to throw some light on the problem, the Newsons analyzed their figures on bed-wetting in several ways. They found a link with social class: 18% of middle class children wet their beds, while 30% of the working class children did. However, explanations for this connection were elusive. They examined the use of physical punishment as opposed to explanation, general neatness and tidiness, and convenience of toilet facilities. In none of these was a statistically significant difference found. No answer could be given.

Many people have assumed that there is some connection between bed-wetting and dreaming. In fact, the wetting usually occurs in the first part of the night, most often at the end of a period of stage 3 or 4 sleep and a shift to stage 1 or 2. In other words, it does not occur in REM sleep and so cannot be triggered off by dreaming. Of course, if the child is wet and then begins to dream the wetness may affect the content of the dream. It is certainly not the other way around.

Another cause that keeps on being suggested is that the bed-wetting child has a small bladder and is physically incapable of holding a nighttime's collection of urine. Such ideas have been "proved" by giving such children a drink of a known amount of fluid and seeing when they need to go to the bathroom as compared with non-wetting children. The fact that the wetters go quicker may mean nothing more than they are more anxious about bladder-emptying than their drier friends. Such "proof" may not be proof at all.

There continue to be many different theories, and whenever a subject has so many suggested answers you can be pretty sure that none of them is completely correct. In particular, psychiatrists and psychoanalysts have had a field day with bed-wetting. Saying that wetting the bed is an act of subconscious aggression against the mother is insupportable, and probably nonsense. Nonetheless, if anyone who believes this theory chooses to challenge me, there is no way that I can prove him wrong. That is the delight of psychoanalysis. Even to doubt what they say can be taken as further proof that they are right, as the doubter is, in their minds, motivated by his own subconscious attitudes. To argue with a psychoanalytical mind is to submit oneself to "Heads I lose, tails you win."

One theory that I do find interesting suggests that around the age of three there is a critical period for becoming dry at night. J.W.B. Douglas, in a review of the problem in 1967,[2] found that there was a correlation between bed-wetting at four-and-a-half years and the number of stressful events which occurred when the child was two or three, such as illness, operation, and separations from the family.

Others suggest that, in a given child, wetting at age three may be due to a cause such as simple delayed maturation, at four it may be due to anxiety, and at five to having missed the chance of learning at the critical time around three.[3] Later still anxiety may be a problem—this time anxiety about the enuresis. There is a degree of sense in this sort of argument, but I remain impressed by Werry, who examined the possible causes and concluded that there was no single obvious cause and that easy over generalizations are best ignored.[4]

The negative theories have produced some useful information. Enuresis is definitely not evidence that a child is neurotic. A neurotic child may be enuretic. It does not follow that the enuretic is neurotic—though in the past many doctors and parents did make the mistake of saying that it does.

Physical causes are also unusual, particularly in the child who is only wet at night. It is difficult to understand how something physically wrong with the bladder, kidneys, or rest of the urinary system can cause problems only at night. Children who have daytime problems with urination as well do need closer assessment.

Among the mythical reasons for bed-wetting that get passed down from mother to mother are such supposed causes as a long foreskin, pinworms, and excessive deep sleep. This last one is interesting. There is almost as much evidence to say that it isn't important as evidence to prove that it is.[5] Some deep sleepers are bed-wetters and some are not.

It is probably fair to conclude that among possible causes for enuresis are delayed maturation, social factors, emotional factors and, rarely, physical causes. Whatever has caused the problem, the area of most concern to the parent is what should be done about it. Before considering medical management, it is very interesting to see how parents themselves try to cope.

The Newsons found that parents tried punishment, threatening and shaming the child, bribery, praising success, showing kindness, offering a new bed, playing the whole thing down, and becoming angry. Every method works for some children sometimes. In other words, after trying any of these approaches some children become dry, though this does not prove cause and effect. Other parents had tried each of these approaches in turn and had failed every time. What does seem likely to help is a change in technique. Maybe it is the change that helps, rather than the actual method. Children could get bored with one method, and trying another revitalizes their interest.

The most common advice that these parents had received about the problem was to cut down on drinks at bedtime. This can make the problem worse, as the child goes to bed thinking about drinks in the same way as a person thinks far more about food when on a diet than when not on a diet. Such an approach is bound to fail. There is definitely no evidence to prove that giving a child a drink at bedtime is a cause of bed-wetting.

The other piece of advice that the parents often received was to try picking the child up at night. I am far from happy about this approach. Commonsense says that unless the child is completely awake he will still be urinating in his sleep and so is not learning a new skill, and forcibly to wake a child in the middle of the night seems to me to be punitive in the extreme. It is of course perfectly reasonable to carry your child to the bathroom or to the potty while he is still asleep as long as you realize that this only serves the quite natural purpose of saving you the extra trouble of washing yet more sheets. It does not go any way toward curing the problem in the long run.

As far as my two children were concerned, "bribery" worked like a dream with Katy. When she was two-and-a-half she asked us if she could have a grown-up, pretty nightgown. We told her that she could as soon as she was out of diapers, as they weren't really suitable under a nightie. To our astonishment, the very next morning she came into our bedroom defiantly waving her dry diaper. Christopher, however, was totally disinterested in the whole business. Some nights he was wet, and some he was dry. We were less bothered too; perhaps because we had invested in a new washing machine which made it easy to wash the sheets. Eventually, sometime around four years, we realized Christopher had been dry for a week and had left his diaper off. For the next few months excitement made him wet, but these occasions gradually got fewer and fewer.

Assuming you haven't been so lucky and you consult your doctor about a bed-wetting child, what will he do? To begin with he will want to know if your child has ever been dry. If he hasn't, the problem is known as primary enuresis. If he has, and has subsequently become wet, it is secondary enuresis. For the latter he will ask questions about the time that the wetness started. Was there a new brother or sister? Was there a car accident or some other trauma? For all enuretics he will also ask questions about daytime bladder control.

Having found out as many details as possible about the problem, a physical examination and a urinalysis will follow. There is no need for complex examinations such as kidney scans and X-rays in the huge majority of cases, but the urine examination is essential to ensure that there is no infection present or any evidence of kidney disease. Following the urinalysis, the doctor will attempt to explain the problem, to reassure, and to put it into perspective. For the parents such a discussion can often make them realize that their child is more normal than they thought, and if their fears about underlying medical or psychiatric causes can be put to rest, the whole topic can become far less stressful. This in itself can improve the emotional climate of the house around bedtime and be enough to cure the problem.

The most important advice the doctor can give is to be positive. Praising dry nights, and ignoring wet ones, is generally much more effective than punishing the wet ones. This technique is often used in star charts. These are charts marked with the days of the week on which the child marks his dry nights. A typical chart involves the child sticking a blue star in the relevant space each time he has a dry night, with a gold star being used for three dry nights in a row. It is essential that the child himself do the sticking. He then has to present it to the doctor after a few weeks to show how he has done, and the doctor will reinforce the child's improvement by praising the dry nights. The scheme is continued until the child has had two months almost completely dry. The method is totally free of side-effects, and I still find myself astonished by how successful it can be. The praise can even be accentuated by sheer bribery. The parents may offer a small gift for three gold stars. I personally don't advise this until it is clear that the child is improving anyway, when the extra praise can speed up the process. For the child who is not improving, to fail to get the gift can reinforce his own views of his inadequacy.

The other simple treatment that some doctors advise in addition to the star chart is the "bladder drill." This is not a horrific instrument reminiscent of the dentist, but a method of training the bladder. The doctor explains to the child that the bladder is simply a muscle and, like any other muscle, it can be trained and strengthened. The child is instructed that when he next urinates he is to stop in midstream and count as far as possible before beginning again. He is encouraged to try to count to twenty and told that when he can do this he is more in command of his bladder. This control can therefore be continued through the night. I doubt whether this is anything more than a clever form of suggestion, but it can work. (Incidentally, it is said that if you should enter the toilets of certain children's hospital outpatient departments, you will find a chorus of little boys desperately trying to count to 20.)

Mention of suggestion also brings to mind the use of hypnosis. In hypnosis the child is encouraged repeatedly to believe that he will stay dry at night, and enthusiasts claim an impressive record of successes.[6] It is really only of use in children over age eight. Other suggestions can also be used to encourage the child. For instance, he can be reassured that the wetness does not really matter, thus lowering the stress level and that he will be able to wake up if he does need to urinate. The problem with hypnosis is that it is time-consuming, and skilled practitioners are few; as yet it is available to relatively few. The advantages are many; it is kind, safe, and is designed to allay fears and boost the child's image of himself—an image that the bed-wetting may have considerably upset.

Should star charts, the bladder drill, and advice all fail, then what comes next? In the past, fascinating methods have been tried. The first medical book on the topic in the English language was Thomas Phaer's *Book of Children*. In the section on "Pyssing in The Bedde," the recommended treatments involved such ingredients as the windpipe of a cock and the claws of a goat. It even recommended "the stones of a hedgehogge poudred." Other treatments over the years have included applying stinging nettles to the penis, putting an inflated bag in the vagina and, in Nigeria, the tying of a toad to the penis so that it croaks when the child urinates and so wakes him up!

Modern treatments are somewhat different, although they may seem quite bizarre two hundred years in the future. There are two main approaches. Many doctors use medication, in particular the group of drugs known as the tricyclic anti-depressants. The best known of these are imipramine and amitryptylline, which are marketed around the world under various names. While how they work is uncertain, it has nothing to do with their being a treatment for depression. More likely they work by making the muscle controlling the emptying of the bladder less sensitive. Used by themselves they can often produce a fairly rapid end to bed-wetting, which returns almost as soon as they are stopped. However, if combined with methods like star charts, they can be far more beneficial. Their use is gradually becoming less frequent and tends to be reserved for occasions such as school trips abroad, or when a mother is becoming absolutely desperate. They may also be used when a child has totally lost confidence that he will ever become dry. The reason for their falling out of favor is simple: if an overdose is taken, they can be extremely dangerous. Childproof containers and parental vigilance can lessen the risk, but for there to be any risk at all may not be acceptable when one is treating a harmless, albeit often infuriating, condition.

Perhaps the modern mainstay of treatment is the enuresis alarm. This consists of a buzzer unit connected by a flexible wire to a metal pad in the child's bed. The unit is battery operated and completely safe. When a small amount of urine is passed, the alarm goes off and wakes the child, stopping urination immediately. The child can then go to the bathroom normally. Gradually, after several nights of being woken, this reflex action becomes automatic and the child wakes before the alarm. On the average, being woken by the alarm fifteen times is enough to stop the bed-wetting.

The success rate varies, but one medical source claims that 80% of bed-wetters will be cured in a period varying from one week to six months, with an average of three-and-a-half to four months.[7] It is not an easy method to use, and it is essential that it is properly understood by the parents. Crowded homes, shared rooms, and very deep sleeping children make the method more awkward, but still possible. And success can still be achieved in these circumstances.

Once a child has been dry for about three weeks the method can usually be discontinued. There are those who have criticized the method for being illogical, saying that if after using the alarm the child wakes up to urinate then the ideal of going through the night dry and asleep has not been achieved. In fact, even though the alarm initially leads to the child waking to go to the bathroom, within a few weeks this waking usually stops and the night is undisturbed.

Recently a very small electronic alarm has been introduced which is far less cumbersome than the older models. According to a medical journal article, it is cheaper than earlier alarms, and very successful. Children who had tried both the old and new alarms greatly preferred the mini-version, which has a sensing pad applied directly to the underpants. The great advantage of this is that normal nightclothes can be worn, in contrast to the advice given with the older units that pajama bottoms should be left off. It is odd to think that this is nothing more than an electronic version of the old African method of tying a toad to the penis!

Finally, yet another drug has been evaluated for the treatment of enuresis and has been found to be highly effective.[9] The drug DDAVP, or desmopressin, is inhaled at bedtime. This drug is an antidiuretic hormone and has a direct effect on the kidneys, reducing the production of urine. It works very effectively and the results of a trial in Israel were impressive, but sadly, stopping the treatment resulted in a return to wetting. The drug is expensive, and I cannot believe that it will find a significant place in everyday management. It is only one of a long list of treatments that date back to the Ebers Papyrus in 1550 B.C. It certainly won't be the last.

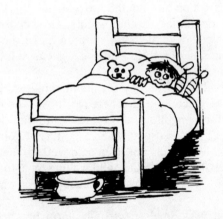

• 9 •

Special Cases

The sleep problems of the handicapped, the gifted and the hyperactive

Aᴵᴵ children may have any of the common problems already described, but certain groups have additional problems or have an increased incidence of particular sleep disturbances.

THE HANDICAPPED

The child with poor hearing appears to be especially prone to night waking and settling problems. In 1977 a comparison was made between 68 children with impaired hearing and a group of children with normal hearing.[1] Both groups were found to go to bed at the same time and to have the same overall length of sleep, but the deaf children took almost twice as long to get to sleep.

Children who are blind or who have some other form of major visual handicap can also have particular difficulties at bedtime. Many of their parents report problems, and most assume that this is because the child cannot perceive the darkness that usually heralds bedtime. While this would seem a possible explanation, children are far more sensitive to the world than this simplistic approach allows. They can tell when it is bedtime because of the different emotional atmosphere at home, the arrival home from work of the breadwinner, and even the obvious cue of changing television and radio programs. The difficulties are more likely to be bound up with the fact that blind children are often not quite as physically active and busy as other children, and so may well be less tired. Naturally, there is no reason why visually handicapped children should not have any of the sleep problems experienced by their sighted counterparts.

The mentally handicapped are a group with their own specific problems. Children with Down's Syndrome, for instance, can often be very restless during the night, even if they are asleep. This restlessness can lead to their kicking off their blankets, which is in itself not unusual and in other children is not important. However, these children have a relatively inefficient autonomic nervous system which results in very poor control of their body temperature, and so the kicking off of blankets in a cold bedroom can be dangerous.

Poor body thermoregulation may be the cause of their restlessness in that they may feel particularly hot on going to bed. Feeling hot may make them kick their blankets off, and as they were hot immediately before this happened, the skin blood vessels can be dilated, leading to even greater heat loss. Evidence exists that this heat loss can increase their chances of developing throat and chest infections. Down's Syndrome children are more susceptible to infection even at the best of times as their immunological system is relatively inefficient.

Many other Down's Syndrome babies are very much the opposite of sleepless; they sleep excessively. This should be discouraged whenever possible as they can clearly receive no stimulation when asleep and it is only when stimulated that they can develop in any significant way.

Down's children can suffer exactly the same problems of restlessness and sleeplessness as other children, and management should be based on the same principles as those discussed elsewhere. A word of warning, though. Down's children are even more creatures of habit than other children. Changes in routine do not come happily to them. The practice of bed-sharing is almost certainly not a good idea with these children. The habit of being in bed with a parent, not to mention the attraction of the warmth they enjoy compared to the cold when they leave it, can be very difficult to break. I know of one case of a 30-year-old man who is still sleeping with his brother and stepsister. It is wise to avoid bed-sharing as a method of coping with sleep problems in Down's Syndrome children.

Mentally handicapped children may suffer from head-banging, which is by no means specific to the mentally handicapped but tends to be more prolonged and more frequent with them. This and other problems have frequently been dealt with in the past with drugs, and there is little doubt that behavioral techniques can also be extremely effective.[2]

GIFTED CHILDREN

Gifted children tend to have problems too. One of the most common about which parents write is the limited amount of sleep that their babies and toddlers require. The problem seems to arise because the children need far less sleep than do their parents, and the parents subsequently get doubly exhausted. It is bad enough not sleeping at night, but worse still when trying to cope with an inquisitive child who constantly demands attention and stimulation. While not all above average intelligence children sleep less than average, (and sleeplessness does not prove that a child is highly intelligent) there does seem to be some connection in many cases.

The abilities of some gifted children are quite remarkable. One mother wrote of her child who was not only talking in long fluent sentences by sixteen months old, but was playing chess by two-and-a-half years. She found that his sleep always improved dramatically when he was mentally stimulated. Before the age of three her child learned to read and promptly began to sleep through the night. This lasted for about six months. She then taught him to write, and even though his sleep had again become very disturbed, it rapidly improved. She became certain that he needed new mentally stimulating activities to encourage him to sleep through the night. He rarely goes to sleep before 11:30, but reads quietly to himself up to this time and then sleeps right through the rest of the night.

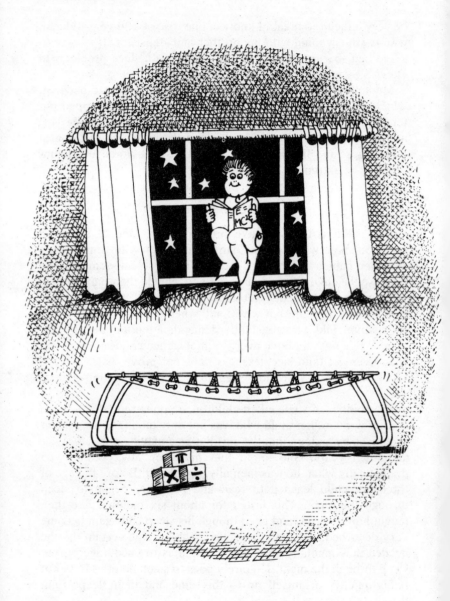

This experience is not unique. An official of a gifted children's association wrote to me of her experiences, and I quote from her letter. "I have been contacted many times by parents who are going through the same sort of difficulties as we experienced, with the same lack of understanding, sympathy, or constructive advice from pediatricians, and I have, in several cases, advised the parents to mentally stimulate their very young children. This invariably worked—the children's sleeping patterns became more normal, and the family's sanity returned."

The truly gifted child clearly has a major problem with sleep, and it has often been said that the child who does not sleep as much is brighter and more intelligent than average. Kind sympathizers tend to say this as some form of consolation. It always used to cheer me up too, to think that my two were such pests because they had superior minds. It is, of course, possible that the child who is awake longer than average has more stimulation and more time to learn, but there does not seem to be any real evidence that sleepless children are the brightest ones.

HYPERACTIVITY

This term covers the child who is physically and mentally restless with boundless energy. These children are impulsive, distractable and excitable. They don't sit still, they talk a lot and sleep very badly. They are totally exhausting for their parents.

However, the diagnosis of hyperactivity is not as clear-cut as that. Some authorities dispute whether such a condition exists as a separate clinical entity. It is interesting that two of the 20th century's leading child care books barely touch on the subject. In Dr. Benjamin Spock's *Baby and Child Care* the subject gets less than a page. Hugh Jolly's *Book of Child Care* does not even mention it. Hyperactivity is, however, dealt with in quite considerable length in Schrag and Divoky's book *The Myth of the Hyperactive Child*—a title which concisely gives the author's views.

I do not wish to here enter the debate on hyperactivity, but it is interesting to note that it is much more common in the United

States than in Britain—a difference that probably reflects doctors' attitudes rather than children's health. Many American doctors believe it is due to "minimal brain dysfunction," possibly resulting from such varied causes as birth trauma, food allergies, and unspecified vitamin deficiencies. Treatment, sometimes involving drugs, is aimed at correcting whatever is seen to be the underlying problem.

In 1973, in California, Dr. Ben Feingold proposed that salicylates, artificial flavoring and food coloring was causes of hyperactivity. He produced two highly successful books advising diets and ways of avoiding these substances, and there did appear to be much anecdotal evidence to support that a diet free of these substances helped. However, in 1980, Frederick Stare and his colleagues from the Department of Nutrition at the Harvard School of Public Health and the American Council on Science and Health in New York, extensively reviewed and reassessed the subject. They concluded that, although the subject is clearly in its infancy, diet plays at most a very minor role.[3] Attitudes and opinions on this subject vary enormously. It is difficult to know who is right, and yet it does seem important to retain a reasonably open mind.

The British view of hyperactivity is rather different. It is clear that while some hyperactive children may have some degree of physiological impairment to the brain, the great majority do not. The problem for this majority is therefore often seen as a behavioral one, with as many causes as there are patients. After other potential causes—such as the side-effects of drugs, or mental retardation are excluded, the family setting must be considered. Is there an imbalance of activity levels between various members of the family, as one author proposes.[4] Is the child simply reacting to not having the chance to exert himself without any inhibitions? Are there other causative anxieties and tensions in the family? There is no doubt that much research is required.

There is equally no doubt that extremely overactive children are no figment of their parents' imagination. As one mother wrote to me, "If you doubt they exist, you try having mine for a week."

Help can certainly be at hand, whether via drugs or psychiatric therapy—particularly behavior therapy. One study of behavior therapy reported an improvement within four to six weeks.[5] The treatment included teaching parents how to handle their child in a way that would eliminate or alter their unacceptable behavior. For example, the child was made to sit for longer, and more often, than he would normally. These times were gradually extended until the child's behavior was more like his less overactive brothers and sisters. It sounds too simple, but it worked. Behavior therapy techniques (see Chapter 11) can be applied to sleep problems in the hyperactive as well as in "normal" children.

Support groups can often help by making parents feel less alone. As a member wrote, "To be told that there was a reason for his frightful behavior helped a little, but did not solve the problem. After two-and-a-half years of sleepless nights it was a relief to discover that it was not my fault."[6]

Hyperactivity, whatever it is, does cause sleepless nights, but the huge majority of sleepless children are not hyperactive. Nevertheless, the conclusion that the problem is not always the parents' fault can still come as a considerable relief.

A potentially important spin-off from the research into hyperactivity may be of relevance to sleepless children who are not actually hyperactive. One of the chemicals that has been suggested to have an adverse effect on some children is a dye called tartrazine. A small proportion of people are sensitive to this dye, although the usual reaction is an actual allergy. A number of parents have found that if they omit it from their children's diet, in particular from food and drink taken immediately before bedtime, their children sleep better. Orange drinks, a bedtime favorite, contain tartrazine, and many parents have reported an improvement when they changed to water or milk.

Tartrazine is slowly being abandoned by many manufacturers, but a close scrutiny of product labels should help tell you if it is still included. In the U.S. it is listed as FD&C yellow dye #5. A ruling is currently pending from the FDA to eliminate tartrazine from all products, except those that are used topically. Indeed,

Wyeth Laboratories has eliminated tartrazine from its product Phenergan, which is an antihistamine often used by parents to help their children sleep.

The problem with any discovery like this is that many parents and doctors become over-enthusiastic about it and blame it for almost all sleep disturbances or other similar chemical sensitivities. At the same time, other people will reject it out of hand as being an exceptionally unlikely cause of problems. My suggestion is that if all else has failed, it might be worth excluding food and drink that contain this orange dye from your child's evening meal and drinks. In a couple of weeks you will know if it makes any difference or not.

A great deal more research is needed in the area of chemical sensitivities, and until properly validated studies have been carried out, the subject is going to remain one of intense controversy.

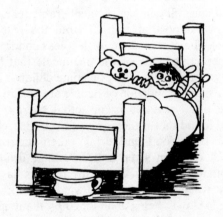

PART

· ▌▌▌ ·

OTHER POSSIBILITIES

· 10 ·

Bed-sharing

Most people have a very clear idea of what a normal, happy, healthy household should look like during the hours of sleep. The parents are tucked up together in bed, and the children are fast asleep either in a room together or, when circumstances permit, in their own individual bedrooms. The children's rooms are warm and comfortable, even the bedding and the wallpaper is cheerful and colorfully coordinated. In all, it is a picture of domestic bliss.

This is such a common vision of affluent Western life in the late 20th century that we tend to assume that it is the only way of organizing sleeping arrangements. Such is our desire for conformity that, should someone find that this system does not work, the reaction is often not pleasure or relief at finding an alternative, but guilt at not following the "normal" methods.

One mother named Judy wrote to me of her feelings about her son. "We had made him this beautiful nursery—cheerful primary colors and patterns everywhere—and he hated it. Every time we put him to bed he screamed. We tried everything: warm room, warm crib, rocking him to sleep, putting him into the crib awake, a musical mobile—all to no avail. Every night we had a screaming match. Eventually, in desperation, though feeling very guilty, we put him into bed with us! Peace—a whole night without a disturbance! Mind you, clinics, doctors, and friends told us what a

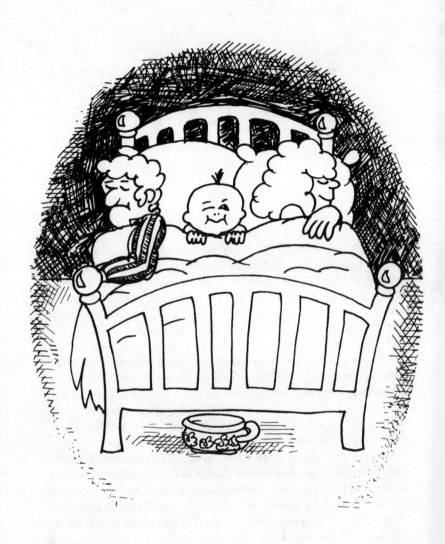

terrible mistake we were making. I reckoned that if it gave us some peace it was worth it, but I felt so guilty and so worried. Would it harm him? I had to know."

Judy need not have worried. Sleeping apart is a relatively new development in human evolution. At many other stages of history, and in other cultures today, the normal arrangement was for the whole family to sleep together. Incidentally, in almost every species other than man, the young sleep with their mother. Yet again, "experts" have declared that there is only one satisfactory way of caring for a child and as a result have caused intense worry for those who want to do otherwise.

Before considering the concept of bed-sharing in detail, I must stress one point very firmly. I am not suggesting that you *should* try bed-sharing if your child does not sleep. What I am saying is that you should do what *you* think is right and best, not what I think is best, nor what anyone else advocates. All I want to do is show some of the advantages and disadvantages and leave it to you to reach a decision. It is worth stating, however, that there is little doubt that many parents have found this practice the solution to their children's sleep problems. I received more letters quoting bed-sharing as a success story than any other solution.

If there were such creatures as child care advisers in the 15th century, then they would have suggested that the child should sleep with his mother at least until the age of two. This was the normal pattern, and according to Tine Thevenin, who has written on the subject at length in her excellent book *The Family Bed*, the 16th century saw the development in England of the Trinity bed.[1] This consisted of a large bed in which the immediate family slept, with two smaller beds called trundle beds kept underneath it and rolled out at bedtime. The trundle beds were for the servants and more distant relatives. One can only hope that there was adequate ventilation for such a mass of sleeping bodies, particularly when considering the relative lack of bathing facilities in those days.

Times changed, and by the 18th century many clergy were pronouncing that it was indecent to go to bed with any other person, and even children were advised to conceal their bodies from one another. Indeed, it is striking that even nowadays many of the euphemisms for sexual activity do not mention sex, but simply sleeping arrangements. To say that someone "went to bed with" or "slept with" someone else usually implies that sleeping was far from their minds.

The 19th century saw the really big change in attitudes toward bed-sharing. The wealthy classes had nannies who looked after the children during the day, and in the evening the children were put into their own nurseries. The idea that too much contact with the child would make him weak and overdependent developed and held sway for far too long, persisting in some people's minds today. In the 1976 edition of *Baby and Child Care,* Dr. Benjamin Spock said that he thought it a sensible rule never to take a child into the parents' bed.

From the 19th century on, Western society has in general pursued the ideal of a separate room for each member of the family. When it works, it is an admirable system. However, while the Western world has separated parents and children overnight, many other societies—particularly in the East—have retained the very ideas that we have rejected. Today, in the West, more and more people are returning to the idea of having their babies in bed with them and we are turning full circle; other cultures have avoided this trauma by following their age-old traditions throughout. It makes one question our concept of progress. Margaret Mead, the internationally respected anthropologist, said, "The fact that co-family sleeping occurs regularly in many human groups, as it does among ours even though the social code is opposed to this practice, is highly significant, and points to a stubborn human characteristic which is worth following up."[1]

There are practical disadvantages in parents and children sharing their beds; there are also feared problems that do not actually exist, such as the worry about overlying the child. The thought of a parent rolling over and suffocating the baby has frightened parents for centuries. It is even mentioned in the Old Testament (1 Kings, 3, v19), and as recently as 1977 a child care manual stated: "Young babies should never sleep in their parents' bed, because there is a very real danger of 'overlaying', which means that the parent turns over in sleep and suffocates the baby."[2]

I am sure this is nonsense. What has almost certainly happened is that in the past the tragedy of crib-death or the sudden infant death syndrome has been blamed on overlying. Affecting two to three of every thousand babies born alive, usually aged between two and six months, a perfectly normal baby is found dead in his bed in the morning. If that child is in bed with you, it is a natural reaction to assume that the death was caused by the parent suffocating the child. In fact, there is no difference in the incidence of crib-death in societies or families who sleep together than in those who do not. Films of families asleep in bed together show that if a parent rolls over, the child will adjust its position automatically. This applies from early infancy onwards. Similarly, a parent will roll over instinctively if the child rolls near him. The only time there is a real risk is if the parent is deep asleep from too much alcohol or sleeping pills.

Another common worry is that the child or baby might fall out of bed. However, it appears that parents unconsciously, as a reflex, put their arms protectively around a child as they sleep, and the problem rarely occurs. If it does worry you, you can always rearrange the room so there is furniture or a wall on one side of the bed.

There is one potentially serious hazard that can arise, at least theoretically, from bed-sharing, but it is one which can easily be avoided. Children's beds tend to be colder places than their parents' beds. As a result, children tend to be dressed for bed in very warm clothes. If halfway through the night you take the child into your bed, do take this extra, warm clothing off. In bed with you, the child will need nothing more than light cotton pajamas or a nightgown.

The reason that this seemingly trivial advice is important is that evidence is accumulating showing that some sudden infant deaths may be a result of a rapid rise in the child's temperature. A warmly wrapped child in bed with two adults could easily become very hot very quickly. Please do not let this happen.

Although large numbers of parents find that having their child sleeping with them helps the child rest—indeed this was by far and away the most frequent solution mentioned by my many correspondents—a number of real worries were raised. The most common related to sex. As one writer put it: "Think twice before putting the baby in the same bed as the parents. It is very difficult to have decent sex without waking it up. We solved this by having an adult sized mattress for the baby on the floor, wedged between the bed and the wall. He slept fine there, and we didn't wake him up once!" While not strictly bed-sharing, this compromise worked for them.

Many couples found that their babies were not waking up until two or three o'clock in the morning. By this time any sexual activity was over, and to take the child into the bed then posed no problem. However, if the child is awake from the adults' bedtime, then obviously if you want to have your baby with you the only solution is to alter either the timing or place of your sex life. There is no law that says it has to be conducted at bedtime in bed. Neverthless, one frustrated couple wrote so say that "we knew our three-year-old would come into our room as soon as we became amorous. Children are a marvelous contraceptive. So one evening we were just getting started on the rug by the flickering living room fire when he came in. 'When are you coming to bed?' he asked. "We could have screamed."

Suffice it to say that if your sex life is suffering, or if either of you resent the intrusion of your child, then bed-sharing is not for you. Similarly, if either of you cannot sleep if a child is in the bed because he or she wriggles, snores, or lies sideways, then it is not worth pursuing the idea.

Another very reasonable alternative to full bed-sharing is having the child in a separate bed in your bedroom. This gets around the problem of the child who wriggles, and many families find it an excellent and effective compromise. One family I know gradually moved their child's bed further and further from their own and found that this approach was accepted with no complaints by their youngster. Eventually the child was moved completely from their room and was happy to see this as a further step in his independence. If you cannot tolerate the child in your bed, but can only get a good night's sleep when he is nearby, then this may be the answer.

I have just dealt with the valid reasons for not sharing the bed. However, there is no evidence that bed-sharing can cause the child psychological harm. Occasionally claims are made that only couples with sexual or marital problems share their bed with their child. For example, a writer in the journal of the American Medical Association in 1980 went so far as to state that because most children in our society do not sleep with their parents, "the physician should consider exploring underlying motives with the parents as to whose needs are being served by this arrangement."[3]

An American study in 1974 claimed that bed-sharing is an indicator of a disturbed parental relationship.[5] This much-quoted study suggested that the mother often used the child's presence as a shield against her husband's sexual demands. However, a 1982 study from Sweden disagreed with this; it did not reveal any increase in divorce rates in families who shared beds with four- to eight-year-olds.[6] As the Swedes concluded, "The habit is too widespread among ordinary families for it to serve as a sign that the parents are in the process of separating."

The final worry that concerns parents is that once the child has slept with them then he will never want to sleep by himself again. This need not be a problem. If the idea of returning to his own room can be sold to the child as part of growing up, then the child is often keen to leave the family bed. Some families told me that when they thought the time was right they redecorated the child's room and waited for him to ask to be allowed to sleep there. As one parent wrote, "It worked better than we ever dreamed. We thought he would be sleeping with us forever, and there he was begging to be allowed into his own room. He was so proud of it. He felt so grown up."

Understandably, if the child is forced back to his own room before he wants, or is prepared, to go he may well resist. An ideal time is probably around the age of three or four, but the child who has been in with his parents from a very early age is far more likely to return to his own bed than one who has been taken in later. Even the child who has happily gone back to his own room may still occasionally want to return to his parents' bed. From the moment I entered general practice I could not fail to notice how many children are nursed in their parents' bed, not in their own, when they are sick. Both parents and children realize the comfort and security that comes from such an arrangement.

This understandable concern that the child will never leave the parents' bed is a very common belief. Grandparents, friends and professionals frequently shake their heads and say that to have the child with you is "asking for trouble." In fact, very few children do want to stay in their parents' bed permanently. It is all a matter of using the right sort of persuasion. Explain to your child that having his own bed is part of growing up, as natural a development as brushing his teeth or tying his own shoe laces, and he will happily and proudly accept the idea. If, however, you suddenly and inexplicably tell him that he has got to go to a cold and uninviting room, particularly one that he does not yet think of as his own, then you can expect resistance. After all, you would feel exactly the same, wouldn't you?

I have deliberately devoted a great deal of space to bed-sharing. It is not always the answer, although it has helped a huge number of parents, and it can certainly avoid those dreadful cold nights sitting in a cold room trying to get a child back to sleep—the experience that makes having sleepless children such a burden. When bed-sharing works, it works well. If it suits you, do it and don't feel guilty or worried about it. If it doesn't suit you, then don't feel guilty either. We are all different.

CHAPTER

• 11 •

Behavior Therapy

Some of the more successful results in treating sleep problems in children have been obtained through using behavior therapy.[1] This approach has been adopted by many doctors, psychologists, and support groups. Behavior therapy is a form of treatment in which patients are gradually trained to replace undesirable habits by more desirable ones. The chief difference between this approach and many other types of psychotherapy is that behavior therapists are not particularly concerned with analyzing the cause of a problem. They simply get on and deal with it. A patient with a phobia does not therefore spend a long time attempting to understand why he has a particular fear, but instead learns to conquer it.

Phobias, or irrational fears, are one area in which behavior therapy has excelled, and a brief description of the approach used demonstrates the essential nature of behavioral methods. The patient with, for example, an irrational fear of spiders is gradually taught to accept spiders nearer and nearer to him. Initially he may be petrified by the thought of there being a spider in the next room. By learning simple relaxation techniques and by taking it slowly, he can grow to accept the presence of a spider in the same room—albeit at a distance. The spider is brought nearer and nearer over subsequent sessions, and the patient continues to use relaxation techniques to accept this. Eventually he may well be able to tolerate several spiders crawling over his hand—something that would have horrified him a few weeks earlier.

You can see from this that the essence of the method is to effect a gradual change in the behavior that is causing the problems, and this can be readily adapted to many sleeping problems. Using the behavioral approach makes two assumptions, the evidence for which I have already discussed at some length. The first is that, by the time a problem has developed, the cause is largely irrelevant. What really matters is the problem itself, not whether it was caused by actions by the parents, or anything else. Parents are usually reassured to know that sleep problems are very frequently not their fault, but in practical terms this does not affect management of them.

The second assumption is, as described in Chapter 2, that all babies and children drift through the various phases of sleep each and every night and frequently awaken. The ones who turn over and go back to sleep do not cause their parents any problems. The ones who call out, or get up, do. Treatment is therefore not aimed at preventing them from waking up, but at encouraging them either to go back to sleep or, at the very least, not to wake their parents up.

At the simplest level, behavior therapy is simply commonsense, and many parents will have adopted these techniques without realizing it. The first step is to define exactly what the problem is and what you would consider to be a satisfactory solution. You then make a gradual attempt to shift from the one to the other.

As an example, take the child who will not settle down until eleven o'clock at night and insists on his mother or father being with him. The ideal for the parents might be for the child to be alone in his room at 7:30. The first step is to set up a satisfactory relaxing bedtime routine. Relaxation is essential to most behavior therapies. Initially the child is put to bed at a late hour to ensure maximum tiredness, and then bedtime is gradually—almost imperceptibly—brought forward.

Sometimes the approach can be very simple, as described here, but on other occasions the situation may have become very complicated and seemingly intractable. It is on these occasions that help may be obtained from psychologists or doctors specially trained in a number of well-recognized behavioral techniques. Your own doctor, if he is not trained in these techniques, will be able to put you in touch with someone who is.

The first of these techniques is known as *reinforcement*. This is aimed at encouraging desirable behavior through praise or various minor privileges, and the star charts (see page 118) are an example of this. In *extinction* an attempt is made to eradicate things that the parent is doing which may be encouraging poor sleep. *Shaping* is a gradual alteration of a child's behavior from the unacceptable to the acceptable. The gradual bringing forward of bedtime is a good example, as is the way a parent may be taught gradually to move further and further away from a child while he goes to sleep. *Cueing* is a term that covers teaching the child what cues or signals mean that bedtime is coming, and the adoption of a standard routine helps here. Finally, *fading* is the gradual removal of artificial aids like star charts so the child may settle down more spontaneously.

Some behavior therapists treat phobias such as the spider phobia far more dramatically. Rather than the gradual build-up, they put the patient in the worst possible situation he or she can imagine, such as a small locked room full of spiders, and let them get over the fear as rapidly as possible. Once the patient realizes that the spiders cannot kill him, then the fear lessens. The equivalent of this for sleepless children would seem to be the technique of leaving your child to scream for as long as it takes to go to sleep. However, as we have already seen, for various reasons this particular technique is frequently a failure.

Before considering how you can adapt some of these behavioral techniques to your particular problem, you should know that it has been suggested that the very fact that they work is proof that parental management may be an important factor in prolonging sleep problems.[2] This does not mean that the parents caused the sleep problems, but it does mean that they may be doing something *now* that keeps it going.

An extremely useful way of finding out more about your own problem is to keep a sleep diary.[3] After months of sleepless nights you may no longer be able to see exactly what the problem is and what may be aggravating it. Behavioral techniques, such as a sleep diary, can often work for babies as well as young children. They can at least help the parents structure the way that they cope with the problem, and research has shown such diaries to be potentially very valuable.

For a couple of weeks it is well worth recording your child's sleep pattern in detail. Each day you should record the following:

1. The time your child went to bed.

2. The time he finally settled down to sleep.

3. Evening waking (i.e. waking before your bedtime).
   (a) The time, or times, of waking.
   (b) The reasons, if apparent (i.e. thirst).
   (c) What you did when he awoke.
   (d) The time he went back to sleep.

4. Night waking.
   (a) The time, or times, of waking.
   (b) Possible reasons.
   (c) What you did when he awoke
   (d) The time he went back to sleep.

5. Time of waking in the morning.

6. His mood on waking.
   You can record this numerically. Take a scale from 1 (as miserable as I can imagine) to 10 (as happy and content as I can imagine).

7. Time of daytime naps.

You could draw a large chart like the one below. Alternatively, you could use a notebook or diary.

	SUN	MON	TUES	WED	THURS	FRI	SAT
Bedtime							
Time settled to sleep							
Evening waking (a) Time (b) Reason (c) Action taken (d) Back to sleep							
Night waking (a) Time (b) Reason (c) Action taken (d) Back to sleep							
Morning waking time							
Mood (on waking)							
Daytime naps							

The first and often immensely valuable result of making this record is that you can, possibly for the first time, see the forest for the trees. You may see a very obvious pattern to the waking. You may realize that your child is having a late afternoon nap because you sit him in front of the television set in order to give you a breather while you prepare the evening meal, and that this in turn is causing you to suffer a disturbed evening. A diary may show that on the days he does not have that nap his sleep pattern improves.

The diary may also be of use if it is shown to a professional adviser. Rather than simply stating that "all nights are terrible," the detailed diary may pin-point a time when the parents can adjust what they do to improve the situation. One mother's diary showed that her son, Philip, was waking half-a-dozen times each night and that she immediately took him a drink of milk. She would then cuddle him back to sleep. In fact, she was rewarding him for waking up but had considered the drink and cuddle to be the only way she was ever going to get him back to sleep.

Her adviser adopted a very straightforward behavioral approach. She was told how her behavior was seen by Philip, when he woke, as being preferable to going back to sleep. A previous adviser had suggested that she should let Philip cry, but this had not been a success and made her feel extremely upset and guilty. What did help was to take things one step at a time. First she changed the drink from milk to water. This created a mild complaint from Philip, but he soon accepted it. Next she stopped cuddling him, and instead just held his hand. Subsequent steps included sitting by his bed but not holding his hand, sitting by the door, sitting in the doorway, and finally waiting outside the door. Eventually Philip did not call out for her when he woke up, but simply turned over and went back to sleep.

Other sleep problems can be handled in similar ways. Sometimes the child will settle back to sleep rapidly. On other occasions, especially with some very strong-willed children, it may take much longer. For example, if you are not happy about your child being in your bed, but have somehow let the habit develop, it may take many nights of taking your child back to his room

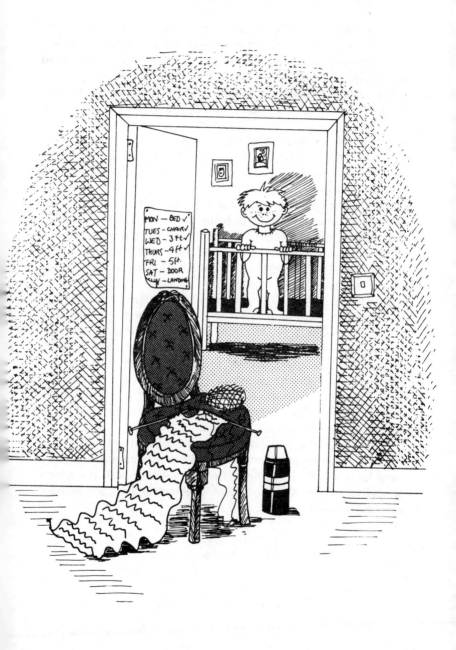

several times a night before he accepts that he has to stay there. Indeed, you may decide that you prefer to wait for him to go back spontaneously. It all depends on how bad the problem appears to be to you.

It is essential when using these behavioral methods that parents do their best to appear calm, relaxed and friendly. This can be difficult if your child has left his room and come downstairs some fifteen or twenty times in an evening. Any parent will feel his or her irritation level rising rapidly. But if you can kindly and firmly take him back to his room, then you are far more likely to succeed than if you show your irritation.

I have talked a lot about the rewards that children can get from their sleeplessness—the fun of being in the heart of the family in the evening, the pleasure of cuddling, the warmth of a parent's bed. However, there is another reward that they gain from sleeping through the nights—the reward of having happy, friendly and relaxed parents the next day!

On occasions, with older children in particular, a system of star charts can be used as a rewarding reinforcement for improved sleeping behavior. I discussed the principle of such charts in the chapter on bed-wetting; in essence it consists of a simple diary chart which the child himself marks with stars when he has achieved a set goal, such as staying in his room throughout a night. This form of positive reinforcement is far more effective with a majority of children than is the negative "I'll wallop you if you make another sound" approach.

Even if you do not intend to follow a full behavioral program, I would strongly recommend that you keep a sleep-problem diary for at least a week. It can be immensely valuable both as a means of understanding your particular problem and as a guide for anyone you might consult.

• 12 •

Sleeping Drugs

Karen was twenty-two. Married for three years, she said she could never remember feeling so desperate. To use her own words, she was shattered. For seven months Michael, her baby, had woken up at least five times every night. Every time he woke she got up to see him. She started every day exhausted; she ended every day frustrated. Her husband slept peacefully through the nights and could not accept that there was a problem. Karen's interest in sex had completely evaporated—she was simply too tired.

It was the sexual problem that finally drove her to the doctor. Her husband had made it clear that if she didn't "sort herself out," he would feel justified in seeking satisfaction elsewhere. She poured out her problems to the doctor. It was clear that there were immense difficulties in this relationship and that they needed attending to. Nevertheless, Karen was simply too tired even to begin the long process of readjusting. Her doctor explained to her that it was no wonder she was exhausted, and that her husband was going to have to share their problems and appreciate that her sexual disinterest was not simply because she was not attracted to him. Not only that, he told her that her feelings of anger and frustration were totally understandable. What she really needed was sleep, and the doctor provided effective therapy for Michael

149

to get five nights of almost guaranteed sleep. The treatment worked. Her son slept and—more importantly—Karen slept too.

About two weeks later she returned to the doctor. She told him that by then she felt like a totally different woman. She had had her hair done and was able to sit and discuss calmly and rationally with her doctor how she should cope in the future with the sleep problem and with her marriage. When she wrote to him to describe her experiences she went on to say, "The funny thing is that after five nights of blissfully undisturbed sleep with the medicine, Michael started waking again when it was stopped. It somehow didn't matter half as much, though. I was rested, and I could see the matter in perspective. I had even managed to talk to my husband about it. I think he finally understood how bad I had felt when he saw how much good the sleep did me. I don't want to have to give Michael the medicine again, but it's good to know it exists."

Karen's story illustrates perfectly many of the advantages of using drugs in the treatment of childhood sleep problems. Incidentally, in this chapter I am only considering the use of hypnotic—or sleep inducing—drugs. Drugs used in the treatment of pain, itching, and the like have been considered earlier (see Chapter 4).

Most doctors will claim to be against the use of drugs in dealing with sleep problems. Indeed, a majority of parents declare themselves reluctant to resort to them. With this being the case, one cannot help but wonder how it is that in one study published in 1977, 25% of a group of first-born children under study had received night sedation by the age of eighteen months.[1]

There are two people for whom drug treatment might be used— the parent or the child. Treating the parent, usually the mother, with a hypnotic drug may present considerable practical problems. At least one parent needs to be able to wake for the child, if necessary, and this may prove tricky if one parent normally sleeps deeply and the other has treatment. In a one-parent family the sedating of the only parent is clearly unwise. Indeed, the majority of parents are very reluctant to receive therapy themselves. There are two occasions when it is justified. The first is when one parent is totally exhausted from insomnia and the other parent is prepared, and able, to wake for the child if needed. The other occasion is to help stress to the normally undisturbed partner how seriously the doctor and patient (the other parent) both view the problem. For a mother to be able to tell her husband "the doctor insists that I take these and get some sleep" may, just may, make him realize that there is a major problem.

Sleeping tablets obviously have many disadvantages and problems which have been adequately made known in recent years. However, most of these do not apply if the treatment is restricted to four or five days at most.

Treating the child with a medicine to help him sleep has both advantages and disadvantages. There are those people who will advise medicine for every child who does not sleep; there are others who feel that it is a total disgrace and that it should never be resorted to. The truth, of course, lies somewhere between the two extremes.

The chief reason for using such treatment is to break the vicious cycle of poor parental sleep which causes tiredness, which causes short tempers and tension, which causes domestic problems, which then cause anxieties which prevent sleep. Drug treatment is no substitute for counseling, discussion, and other simple measures, but there is little doubt that parents may become so tired that they are unable to sort out the problem adequately for themselves. After a couple of nights sleep they may be sufficiently rested to be able to face the problem again and to work out ways of dealing with it.

Using medication can give everyone a breather and a chance to get enough strength back to consider the problem in other ways. Many authorities refer to drugs as having a use in terms of breaking a bad habit and starting a good one.[2] This can certainly apply in the short-term. A child whose sleep pattern has been disturbed by some occurrence like an accident or hospitalization may well be eased back into his normal pattern by a brief course of treatment. For children with longer-term problems of an unknown cause, it might be worth trying a course of medication for four or five nights. In most cases there will be no change in the sleep pattern, but in a small proportion medication will be the answer.

Sleeping medication has a number of serious disadvantages. To begin with, it can offer too quick and easy a solution for the doctor who is consulted. Also, it is never a long-term solution, and without some form of counseling the doctor has performed the equivalent of giving a pain killer without beginning to find out why there is a pain.

Secondly, the whole concept of seeking a pharmacological treatment for every problem that a parent faces is unhealthy and unnatural. It should not be necessary to seek a pill for every ill. For a parent to seek such a solution to every child rearing problem is clearly unacceptable. Nonetheless, I cannot go along with those who consider its use a disgrace. One mother wrote to me to say that she was appalled that any doctor would want to "drug my baby into a doped oblivion." To give a parent a few nights rest when she is at the end of her rope may be more of a kindness than this intolerant description suggests.

Many parents do comment that after being given medication their children are generally confused the next day and seem irritable. It is often difficult to know if this is a direct effect of the medication, but it is another reason for restricting medication to a minimum. As one mother wrote to me, "In desperation I once asked my doctor for sedatives. I slept wonderfully, but the next day Simon [her three-year-old] was like a walking zombie. I've never felt so guilty. To think I'd do that to him just so I could get some sleep!"

The other major disadvantage of drug treatment is, in a way, also an advantage. It rarely works for long. After a week or so of treatment it frequently becomes less effective. There is currently never any justification for continuing a drug for more than a week or two. Occasionally parents keep giving medication for months on end, increasing the dose from time to time to keep the child settled down. This should never be necessary, and is self-defeating. It means that other problems, attitudes, and aspects of family relationships and ways of coping are not being looked at suffi-

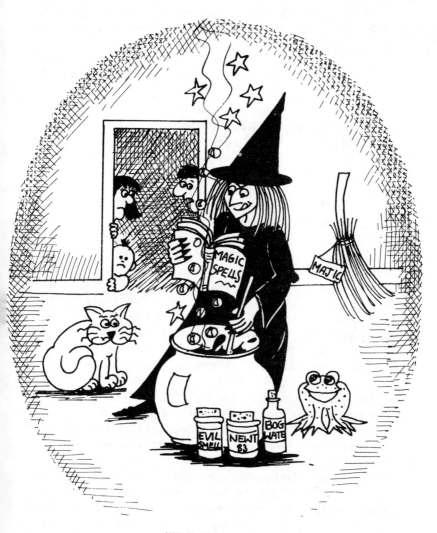

"Well, if this fails . . ."

ciently. In addition, any drug can cause physical side effects if taken long-term. There is also the risk of the undesirable effects on REM sleep that have been caused in adults by the long-term use of hypnotics.

The golden rule when using drugs for children's sleep problems is to restrict their use to a maximum of a week or, very rarely, two, and not to use them continually. Indeed, it can be a great relief to parents to know that such help exists, and some treatments can do a lot of good in lowering anxiety levels without ever leaving the bottle. Drugs should never be used just because a child's sleep does not match some apparent ideal. Such ideals are irrelevant. If your child does not go to sleep when everyone else's child does, and you can adapt your life to cope with this, then there is obviously no need to drug the child because he doesn't fit everyone else's schedules.

If you are going to use drugs it is essential to use them so that they work. Nothing is more damaging to the parents' self-confidence, after having made the decision to use a drug, than for it to let them down. It is very important to use an adequate dose. Many people—parents and doctors—start half-heartedly with a small dose. Not only may this not help, but many sedative drugs paradoxically stimulate in a lower than recommended dose. Children also rapidly become habituated to drugs. If they are given a low dose at the start and this is gradually increased, then the dose that eventually helps may be far greater than the dose that they needed in the beginning. The parents, too, will have become desperate because the promised relief isn't materializing.

It is also important to use the drug at the right time. If a child has a problem of waking at three in the morning, it is often pointless giving the treatment when they go to bed at six or seven in the evening. The hypnotic effect may work during the evening and then wear off by the time it is needed. The time from administering to effect varies from drug to drug and child to child. However, if the problem is one of failure to get to sleep, then medication needs to be given before the child goes to bed so that he is sleepy when he gets there.

There are several different drugs available for use in the management of sleep disorders. It is worthy considering these individually.

Promethazine

Promethazine has for years been a popular drug in helping this problem. Its popularity can be shown by the number of names it goes by in the United States—Ganphen, Quadnite, Remsed, ZiPan, Promine and Phenergan! All are available by prescription only.

It is an antihistamine, and is also remarkably safe. However, safety is never an excuse for not keeping a drug out of a child's reach. In 1962 a two-year-old boy died after taking twenty 10 mg tablets. He was very ill when admitted to the hospital, but the story of overdosage was not known at the time, so appropriate treatment was delayed. I have visited many houses where this medicine was left easily in reach of children. Nevertheless, let me stress that serious side effects with Promethazine are extremely rare. It can, though, cause a dry mouth and stuffy nose.

For use as a hypnotic, the dose again varies with age and size. On the average, infants from six months to a year require 10 mg; one- to five-year-olds need 15–20 mg; and five- to ten-year-olds 20–25 mg.

Chloral Hydrate

This has long been a favorite choice of doctors, but is now less popular than in the past. Ten years ago one pediatrician described it as "the best sedative for babies."[5] It has been particularly popular in the United States and Canada, but has one tremendous disadvantage—it tastes appallingly bitter.

The dosage for children is 30–50 mg per kilogram body weight, up to a maximum single dose of 1 gram. Side effects are again few. Rashes can occur, as can occasional nausea. If used over prolonged periods then dependence can occur, as it does with alcohol or barbiturates—yet another reason for keeping its usage to a minimum.

Chloral does not appear to have any effect on the ratio of non-REM and REM sleep. The antihistamines do reduce REM sleep. However, if—as I cannot stress too often—only short-term usage is adhered to, then this is not a problem.

Chloral is usually only available as a liquid, or occasionally as suppositories. In tablet form it is too concentrated and may cause damage to the lining of the gastrointestinal tract.

In my view, the drug has no advantages over the others available, and its taste makes it unpopular with children. It is available throughout the world under the following names: Aquachloral, Felsules, Kessodrate, and Rectules in the United States; Chloradorm, Chloralate, Chloralix, Dormel, Eudorm and Lanchloral in Australia; and Chloralex, Chloralixir, Chloralvan, Chloratol, Nigracap, and Novochlorhydrate in Canada.

Other Sleeping Drugs

You may be wondering what has happened to all the favorite adult hypnotic drugs. Where are the Seconals and the Dalmanes that most people have heard of? The most common types of sleeping tablet used by adults are in the benzodiazepine group of drugs, as are the tranquilizers Valium and Librium. These drugs have been used in the past for sleepless children, but, according to recent medical reports, "are not considered suitable for use in children." They do still have a possible role in the treatment of night terrors and sleepwalking. Certainly you should never give a child any medication that has been prescribed for an adult.

The barbiturates are no longer acceptable treatments either. As with adults, while they used to be helpful, they have been superseded by the improved newer generation of drugs.

There is one aspect of drugs that I hope will one day cease to be as large a problem as I suspect it currently is. The purchase of cough medicines, and other mixtures containing antihistamines, with the express intention of sedating children seems to be more common than I, for one, ever thought. I am sure that most doctors greatly underestimate the magnitude of this (home cure) side of sleep disturbance. One mother, who was also a qualified nurse and a doctor's daughter, wrote at length about this. "I wonder if you realize quite how many mothers resort to baby-doping in times of desperation? It is quite hard for me to admit this as it sounds like a heinous catalogue of crime to list all the things I have used. To justify it I rationalize that after sleepless nights and restless days I would rather give my children something than end up strangling them through sheer exhaustion. All the things I have given them have either been bought over the counter, or under false pretenses on prescription as cough medicine. The list makes me shudder—Benylin, Tixylix, Vallergan, Phenergan, Actifed, Calpol, Disprin. I can't think of any more, but that's enough, isn't it. I feel so guilty."

"Fortunately," she continued, "I am not desperate very often, but one friend uses something every week, and another has spells of using something every night. Many others admit to fairly frequent abuse of over-the-counter medicines. God knows what others don't admit."

Perhaps greater understanding and acceptance of the stresses caused by repeated sleepless nights will diminish the need for such understandable abuse of drugs. Let us sincerely hope so.

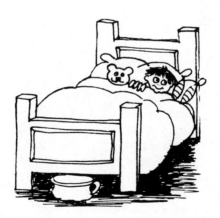

HOW TO SURVIVE

• 13 •

Who Else Can Help?

Despite having considered every facet of sleep disturbance that I have so far mentioned, some unfortunate parents are still going to have problems. The one thing which will help to preserve those parents' sanity, more than anything else, is support and understanding from other people. Obviously the most important person who should offer support is the other parent. Unfortunately, in very many marriages one partner, almost always the husband, sees the problem as being the prime concern of the other. Moreover, many mothers feel guilty if their husband is disturbed at night. In the curious double-think that makes some people, even today, view a husband's work as a "real job" and a wife's as very much a secondary supporting role, there can be much resentment built up because only one of them gets up at night to a sleepless child.

I believe that the duties during the night need to be shared. If the father gets out of bed on some occasions and his wife on others, then at least the annoyance, the sleeplessness, and the cold will be spread more evenly. One mother, who had tried almost every other approach, wrote to tell me that her life had been made bearable when she and her husband split the night into shifts. As she said, "On alternate nights, one of us gets up whenever it is necessary between twelve and six, and the other if

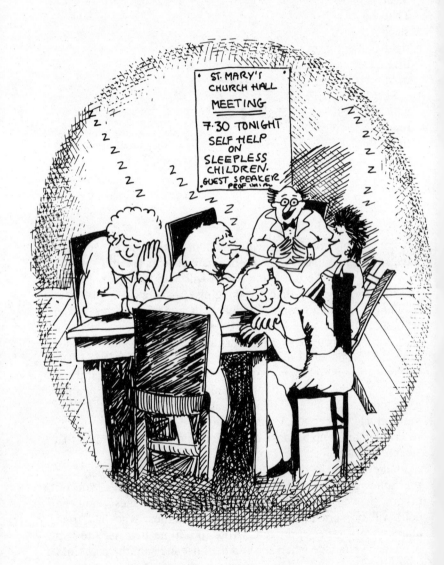

he cries before midnight or between six and eight in the morning. That way we are at least guaranteed six hours of undisturbed sleep every other night." Your work-sharing need not be quite as rigid as this, but it is tremendously helpful for a parent to realize that it will not necessarily be he or she alone on every single occasion.

Such support is denied to the single parent. One organization which aids the single parent has bout seventy independent case reports where the local authority has tried to remove a child from the family. Some of these cases have involved non-accidental injury, and the usual cause has been the inability of the single parent to deal with the demands of the children. This organization feels that, without a doubt, one of the major demands has been the needs of the children during the night. The situation becomes even more stressful because the parent may be unable to meet the child's needs and so the child reacts by requiring even more attention.

Husbands or wives are not the only people who can help each other out. Friends or other relatives often help, although this help is rarely practical. One thing that parents desperately need is understanding. If other people will listen to their problems sympathetically and, above all, believe their nighttime horror stories, then the parents may feel far less alone and inadequate. Many people have support and advice from their own parents, and this is usually most helpful when they too can remember what sleepless nights are like. Other grandparents can be very unsupportive, and reiterate the accusations of "being too soft" or "you've brought it on yourselves" that all parents of sleepless children grow thoroughly sick of.

It helps to have friends with the same problem. One mother wrote, "I found that I only continued my friendship with other mothers who had similar problems. I didn't want to know about good babies!" Many others said that they were very aware that repeated sleepless nights had turned them into bores on the subject. The only people who could stand hearing their stories again were other sufferers.

Sharing one's problems with others can lead to more than just sympathy, important though this is. Other parents may be able to offer advice and survival hints. In a number of places self-help groups have been set up. Some of these are specific to sleep problems, and I know of groups started by parents, by nurses, and by psychologists. These meet regularly and discuss the individual members' problems.

Some of these groups, particularly those that are led by psychologists or others trained in behavior therapy techniques, use behavioral methods in an attempt to improve the sleep pattern of the suffering families. Other groups offer more support than actual advice. Parents share their moans, their problems, and bits of information that they may have heard elsewhere. One mother may have heard a talk on the radio about food additives possibly causing sleep problems, another may have come across a local hospital department with a particular interest in the problem. The information is rapidly passed through such groups to those who most need it. The only danger is that occasionally unproven hypotheses get passed from mother to mother, taking on an aura of "fact" that they do not deserve.

Perhaps the chief advantage of such groups is the easing of the sense of loneliness and incompetence that so many parents feel. One mother told me that she felt much better since she began attending a group since, even though she slept no better, she now felt that she was a "competent and normal mother and not a useless failure." I do hope that this book has the same effect for other parents.

Self-help groups for parents have been set up throughout the United States. The National Self-Help Clearinghouse in New York and the Self-Help Center in Illinois provide information and referrals to self-help groups around the country. Parents Anonymous is a national organization concerned with child abuse. Groups such as these lend a sympathetic ear and offer whatever practical help they can, although most mothers are happy just to know that someone understands and that their feelings are shared by others. Without a doubt such groups can help overcome the isolation and frustration felt by many parents.

A number of self-help groups are assisted by professionals such as doctors or nurses, and there are a large number of medical and paramedical professionals to whom a parent can turn. Sometimes such help can be extremely valuable. Most parents want to be listened to and believed, and even if no practical help is forthcoming they appreciate being given time and sympathy. One mother wrote, "My family doctor has been wonderful. He always lets me talk about my problems, and I keep hoping that he will give me something positive to do that would work. I'm not very hopeful though because I know he still has problems with his five-year-old. If there were an answer, he would surely have found it."

Many other parents are reluctant to ask a doctor's advice. After a seven-page letter detailing a pretty miserable four years, one mother wrote, "All through the time we were going through this ordeal I never thought of seeing the doctor. Although he is a marvelous, sympathetic doctor, I didn't want to bother him with such a trivial complaint. Most babies have some sort of sleeping problem."

There are also, unfortunately, many doctors and nurses who are far from sympathetic. One father summed up his experiences as "Professional help—nil. Doctors laugh, and say it will improve eventually. Ours was most unsympathetic and said she simply didn't believe us when we said how little Peter slept. She said my wife and I must be imagining it."

In a survey published in 1980, parents were asked about the professionals they had consulted about their sleepless children.[1] 45% had found the consultation with their doctor unhelpful. Such a high figure is disturbing. Perhaps it can be explained by a comment in an important research paper on sleep problems that points out that much of what has emerged in research "has not filtered through very effectively." The writers add that, "Our results suggest that some of the advice that comes from these sources (welfare clinics, health professionals, and pediatricians) is not always very helpful and may have little real experience behind it." Such remarks speak for themselves.

One mother did have help from her doctor in an unexpected way. She says she had broken down sobbing in his consulting room. "He told me that if I could not cope he would have to arrange for the children to be taken into care. I couldn't believe it. I told my husband when he got home, and he phoned the doctor and told him we would cope somehow on our own. We have, but I do think the doctor was cruel. Still, since then we have forced ourselves to manage without help, and things seem to be improving."

Apart from sympathy, advice and medication, perhaps the most important help that a medical or paramedical professional can provide is in counseling. An attempt must be made to enable the parents to unravel the complexities of what is happening during the night. The possible causes of sleeplessness and reasons for its continuing need to be explored. Parents may never have considered some of these ideas, and may be able to spot a way of helping themselves. Behavior therapy techniques can also be applied, and I am certain that the use of these will increase over the next few years as more people learn of the principles and uses.

Behavior techniques are often the main therapies in those hospital units which specialize in childhood sleep problems. The development of such clinics is a welcome trend, and the experience they have gained has enabled many psychologists and other workers to set up similar clinics outside the hospitals. The more people who develop an interest in helping this problem, then the better the advice that will eventually be offered.

On rare occasions—to give the parents a much-needed rest—doctors will even admit children to a hospital if they are crying night after night for no apparent reason. This may help to break a vicious circle of sleeplessness for the parents, but it needs to be reserved for the most desperate cases.

Perhaps the most extraordinary therapy I came across in my research was also hospital based. According to a BBC radio report, sleepless children in Russia may be admitted to a sanatorium. When there, they are put to bed while soft classical music is played to them, and they then have electrodes applied to either side of the scalp across which a very low voltage is applied. The system apparently works, but I have been unable to obtain further details from the Soviet Health Service. I find the image it conjures up both bizarre and horrifying, and I certainly do *not* recommend that you experiment along these lines.

An eternity away from the electronic vision that this offers is the age-old practice of homoeopathy. A number of my correspondents told me how they had tried everything else unsuccessfully, and had eventually succeeded with homoeopathic treatment. I find it very difficult to pass judgment on this practice. There is no doubt that many patients claim that it is very helpful, and many doctors practice it very successfully. However, the fact that patients and doctors believe that a treatment is useful does not prove that it is. In my career I have used many treatments that were totally accepted by the medical profession at the time and considered to be the best therapies available. Many of these we now know to be useless. For example, doctors in the recent past used to treat heart attacks with various drugs and three weeks of strict bed rest. The patients got better, and will have been certain that the treatment helped them. I, too, was sure I was helping them. After all, almost all doctors were doing the same thing. Following more stringent analysis and the development of new theories, we now know that the drugs were probably useless in this condition, and the bed rest was positively dangerous. Patients are treated completely differently today, just a few years later. For a doctor and patient to be convinced that a treatment is useful is not good enough, as this example shows. More scientific testing is essential.

Unfortunately homoeopathic treatments are rarely subjected to such stringent tests, and when they are they are seldom seen to be better than "conventional" treatments. This does not mean that they do not work, but I cannot unreservedly recommend them for sleepless children. The best I can say is that they may help, that there are patients and doctors who are very enthusiastic about their use in sleep disorders, and at the very worst they are at least harmless. And this is more than can be said for some of the conventional medicines that doctors use.

The homoepathic principle is to give the child an extremely diluted mixture of a substance, such as caffeine, that would produce insomnia in far greater quantities. The sort of dilutions involved are incredible. It is not unknown for one part of a substance to be diluted with one hundred parts of water, and for this dilution to be repeated thirty times. Arithmetically this dilution would be represented by the fraction 1 over 1 followed by 60 zeros.

The other homoeopathic approach is to determine the individual's own constitutional type, and then use a specific constitutional medicine to help. This is particularly the case with chronic conditions. The physician takes a detailed history and determines exactly what sort of personality profile and physical make-up the patient has, and then selects a therapy to match. For example, an artistic, affectionate, timid person will almost certainly receive different therapy for his migraines than will an outgoing hardworking party-going person. This assessment of the patient as an individual must surely be a good thing, and it is a sad comment on much of conventional medicine that people often complain that they are not treated in this way. Perhaps this is the reason for much of the satisfaction with homoeopathic methods.

The homoeopathic practitioner who treats a sleep problem in a child will therefore consider all the many other, non-drug, aspects of the problem that I have already discussed. These remain vitally important in each and every case.

As for hypnosis, there is little doubt that children under the age of nine are less susceptible than adults and older children.[3] However, for the older child with a sleep problem it may well be worth considering this approach, and most doctors would be able to put you in touch with a reputable hypnotist.

CHAPTER
· 14 ·

Keeping Going

This chapter ignores the child and concentrates on you. How can you best cope with disturbed nights and wake up in the morning sufficiently refreshed to face another day?

Philip, a father of a sleepless three-year-old, expressed feelings that many parents experience. "I don't suppose I really ought to be complaining," he wrote. "Clare probably isn't half as bad as many of the children you have heard about. She only wakes once, or at the most twice, each night but when I have woken up to deal with her I just cannot get back to sleep. The frustration of knowing this will happen often makes me feel unjustifiably angry with her. I know it's not her fault, but I just can't help it."

Anger is a very understandable emotion at a time like this, but unfortunately it inevitably worsens the problem. If you get back into bed seething at the injustice of being blessed with a sleepless child, you are hardly likely to be in a sufficiently relaxed frame of mind to get yourself back to sleep. The parent who is more placid has a considerable advantage here.

There seem to be two ways of ensuring that you will not fall asleep quickly. The first is to lie there fuming about how unfair and unjust the problem is, and the other is by positively trying to go back to sleep. Few activities seem more destined to keep people awake.

Instead of tossing and turning, try relaxing yourself first. This may be achieved by reading a couple of pages of a book or a magazine. A few people listen to soothing music on headphones. Do anything at all to avoid lying there thinking how you cannot sleep and how you may be woken up again soon. If you still feel angry about your child it is worth trying to think of the pleasant, relaxing, and fun times that you have spent together. This usually helps to lessen the irritation, and while you may not start to think of your child as a little angel, he will stop appearing to be the devil he seemed before.

If relaxation is a problem, yoga classes can be very helpful, and there are also some simple exercises that are well worth practicing. These can help almost anybody to unwind. Practice them regularly so that you can use them whenever you feel you are getting tense, and not just to help you sleep. Once you have mastered the art of relaxation you will be able to use it at will, but if you have not practiced beforehand you will find it much harder to achieve a relaxed state.

For one of the most beneficial exercises you need to wear loose clothing and either lie on the floor or a bed. Start by screwing up your face muscles as tightly as you can, and then let them relax. Work through all the face muscles in turn: frowning to tense the forehead, and then relaxing; screwing up the eyes and then relaxing; clenching the jaw and then letting it fall loose.

When you have relaxed the face, next lift up your head and then let it fall gently back. Next relax your shoulders. Start by pressing them down on to the floor or bed and then let them go loose. The arms and fingers are next, and the technique is similar. Hold them out to the side and make them as taut as you can, and then relax them completely. Finally lift each leg into the air for thirty seconds, making the muscles as tight as you can. Then let them suddenly go limp, and drop back to the floor.

When you are practicing, relax the legs, arms, neck, forehead, eyes, and jaw one after the other for about ten minutes, followed by a short period of lying still and loose. Laboratory tests have shown that a period of concentrated relaxation like this can be more beneficial than a standard dose of a tranquilizer, with no side effects and the benefit of being able to use it at will. You will soon be able to climb back into bed, let everything go totally relaxed, and sink back into a restful sleep.

Some people find slow deep breathing very helpful as a means of relaxing. To practice this you simply need to breathe slowly and deeply for a minute at about half the speed you normally breathe. If you feel dizzy, stop. You are probably going too fast. If you can combine slow, deep breathing with relaxation of the muscles you will get even greater benefit.

On a much simpler level, you will find it much harder to get back to sleep if you are cold, or if you have an uncomfortable bed. If you are having problems with your sleep you may find an answer here. There are also many gimmicks such as eyeshades to help you sleep. Try them if they appeal to you. You have nothing to lose but your money.

I cannot possibly deal in this chapter with all the sleep problems that adults can suffer, but only with those that are related to sleepless children. There are several excellent books of advice for adult insomniacs available on the market.

If you refer to Chapter 2, you will see that sleep research has looked into the different quality of disturbed and undisturbed sleep. Disturbed sleep, even if it adds up to eight or more hours in a night, produces more tiredness than six hours of undisturbed sleep. Think about the implications of this. If you can somehow get yourself an undisturbed six hours, then you will cope much better the next day. This is where the sort of sleep rotation mentioned by one couple earlier makes so much sense (see page 161). Divide the nights up with your partner so that if your child wakes each and every night you can still guarantee yourself an undisturbed six hours of sleep, at the very least, on alternate nights. You should get far more rest from this than if you both try to get up on random occasions throughout every night.

If you still find it quite impossible to get enough sleep at night, then try to get a nap during the day. Even if you only get a few minutes of sleep, it can help, and many parents find that the ideal time for this is when there is a pre-school children's program on television. Your child can sit there absorbed by the story and

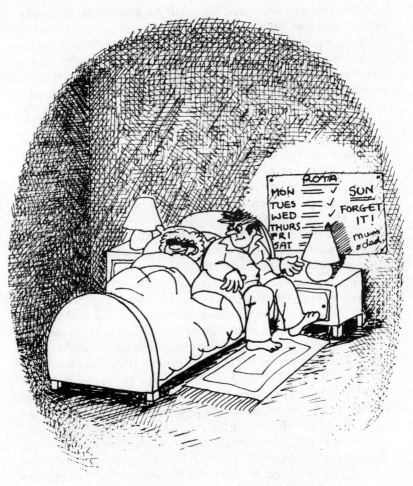

"While you're up, make the tea . . ."

pictures while you grab a few minutes of well-earned rest. Hospital doctors who work long hours and have disturbed nights find that they can keep going by getting what sleep they can when they can. If it works for them, I am sure you can adapt it to work for you.

Finally, if you can become extremely philosophical about losing sleep, you might even find some advantages. By being woken an hour early every day you gain 365 extra hours of potentially useful time every year. Believe it or not, that is equal to more than nine, forty-hour work weeks each year. I don't know how you would spend that extra time, but I certainly found it invaluable. In fact, even though my children no longer have a sleeping problem, I have kept the habit of getting up an hour earlier every day. The extra time was just enough to let me write this book!

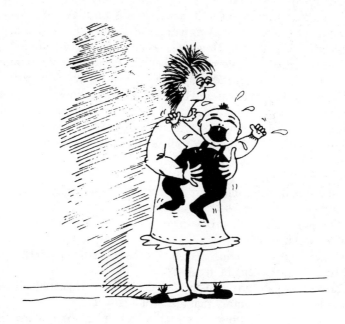

CHAPTER

· 15 ·

Conclusion

When a new baby is born, its parents look on it as tiny, fragile, and helpless. They may even wonder if it will survive the many hazards of childhood. However, after only a few months of sleepless nights, this worry may well be replaced by the parents wondering if they, not the baby, can survive for much longer.

I hope this book has offered both guidelines on how to cope and alternative ways of considering the problem. There are many factors involved, and by now you will have looked at most of the following points, although not all of them will necessarily have been quick or easy to answer.

- Is there really a problem, or are you comparing your child with unrealistic or unnecessary expectations?
- What precisely is the problem?
- When did it start?
- Is there an underlying physical cause, such as eczema or discomfort, that can be treated?
- Can you isolate any causes that could have triggered off the problem, or any factors that are prolonging it?
- Are you yourself doing anything which might be making the problem worse, such as rushing in to the child at his first whimper?

- What advantages does your child get out of waking or not going to sleep?
- Do you get any advantages out of the current situation?
- What effects is the waking having on the family?
- What happens if the child stays with relatives or friends? Does the problem disappear? If it does, you certainly need to explore further what happens when he is with you.
- Can you alter your bedtime routine or your child's sleeping arrangements to help?
- Have you found a solution, but feel guilty about using it?

You will have thought about where you might turn for help, correct and incorrect ways of using medication, and simple conditioning techniques. You should also realize by now how great a problem this can be for very many parents, and you will know that many sleep problems are simply variations within a normal range, rather than an illness requiring treatment. I certainly hope you will not now be feeling guilty about the problem, nor consider that your child is necessarily being naughty or abnormal.

It is quite likely that the sleepless nights will have made you think twice about having more children. There is little evidence that the next child is any more or less likely to have problems, so it remains very much a gamble. If you have decided that some of your problems have been aggravated by your management, then at least you will be better prepared the next time, but this sadly does not guarantee that you will not have one of those babies who is just not a good sleeper. For many parents of sleepless children the thought of the next child never arises. After all, they never have enough time alone together to conceive of the idea, let alone the child.

If you do decide to have more children, and wonder how you can prevent the problem from happening again, then perhaps the most important thing that you can do is adopt a consistent, relaxed bedtime routine, and as consistent a policy on night waking as you can. You may opt for bed-sharing, or for the technique that brought success with your earlier child. With luck the problem will not recur, but as the causes of sleeplessness are frequently beyond our control, this cannot be guaranteed.

Despite everything, a few parents are going to have problems until their child grows out of his sleeplessness. In time, hard though this is to believe, he will stop bothering you at night, even if he does persist in waking up during the night. The older child who sits and reads in his bed or plays in his room when he wakes up causes no problem to anyone. If he needs the rest, he will soon settle down again. As long as you get your sleep, then the time of your life when you suffered from sleepless children will have ended forever.

This is more than just wishful thinking. One doctor that did an extensive survey into children's sleep problems in his practice, found that 40% of children were considered by their parents to have had significant sleep difficulties. The good news is that most of these had stopped being a problem by around their fourth birthday. All problems should cease by their fifth. Hope is in sight. Indeed, one day you may even have trouble persuading your teenagers to get up in the morning.

Sleep well.

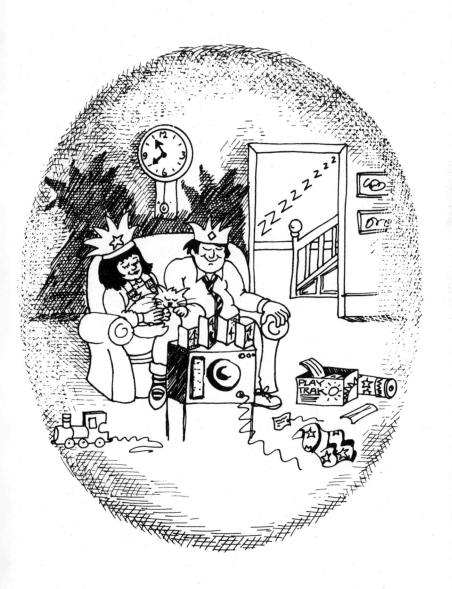

ORGANIZATIONS

◆

National Self-Help Clearinghouse
Graduate School and University Center
33 W. 42nd Street
City University of New York,
New York, New York 10036
212-840-7606

Self-Help Center
1600 Dodge Ave.
Suite S-122
Evanston, Illinois 60201
312-328-0470

Parents Anonymous
22330 Hawthorne Blvd.
Suite 208
Torrance, California 90505
213-371-3501

Parents Without Partners
7910 Woodmont Ave.
Suite 1000
Bethesda, Maryland 20814
301-654-8850

National Association for Gifted Children
2070 Country Road H
St. Paul, Minnesota 55112
612-784-3475

National Organization of Mothers of Twins Club
5402 Amberwood Lane
Rockville, Maryland 20853

La Leche League International
9616 Minneapolis
Franklin Park, Illinois 60131
312-455-7730

American Council of the Blind
1211 Connecticut Avenue, NW
Suite 506
Washington, DC 20036
202-833-1251

Mental Retardation Association of America
211 E. 300 South St.
Suite 212
Salt Lake City, Utah 84111
801-328-1575

National Association for Down's Syndrome
Box 63
Oak Park, Illinois 60303
312-543-6060

Down's Syndrome International
11 N. 73rd Terrace, Rm K
Kansas City, Kansas 66111
913-299-0815

REFERENCES

◆

CHAPTER 1

Sleepless Children—Who Suffers?

1. Jolly, H., *Book of Child Care* (Sphere Books, 1981): 105.
2. Illingworth, C. & Illingworth, R., *Babies & Young Children* (Churchill Livingstone, 1977): 173.
3. Newson, John and Elizabeth, *Patterns of Infant Care in an Urban Community* (Pelican Books, 1976).
4. Richards, M. & Bernal, J., "Why some babies don't sleep," *New Society* (1974) 28: 509-11.
5. Seiler, E. R., "Sleep Problems in Children," *Practitioner* (1972) 208: 271-6.
6. Anders, T., Weinstein, P., "Sleep and its disorders," *Paediatrics* 50: 312-24.
7. Schnedider, C. et al: "Interviewing the Parents" in Kempe, C. H. & Helfer, R. E. (eds.) *Helping the Battered Child and his Family* (Philadelphia & Toronto, Lippincott).

CHAPTER 2

Normal Sleep

1. Parmelee, A. H., "Sleep Cycles in Infants," *Develop. Med. Child. Neurol.* (1969) 11: 794-5.
2. Bax, M., "Sleep Disturbance in the Young Child," *B.M.J.* (1980) 1177-9.

3. Sassin, J., Parker, D., Mace, J. et al, "Human growth hormone release—relation to slow wave sleep and sleep waking cycles."
4. Hartmann, E. L., *The Functions of Sleep,* Yale University Press (1973).

CHAPTER 3

The Sleepless Child—Why Problems Arise

1. Powell, B. W., *Practitioner* (1972) 208: 198-202.
2. Sundell, C. E., *Practitioner* (1922) 109: 89.
3. Strube, G., *Modern Medicine* (Nov. 1981) 19.
4. Richards, M., Bernal, J., "Why some babies don't sleep," *New Society* (28th Feb. 1974).
5. Bernal, J. F., *Develop. Med. Child Neurol.* (1973) 15: 760-9.
6. Moore, T., Ucko, L., "Night Waking in Early Infancy," *Archives of Disease in Childhood* (1957) 333-42.
7. Richman, N., "Sleep Problems in Young Children," *Archives of Disease in Childhood* (1981) 56: 491-3.
8. Chavin, W., Tinson, S., "Children with Sleep Difficulties," *Health Visitor* (Nov. 1980) Vol 53: 477-80.
9. Tizard, J., Tizard, B., "Social Development of 2 year old children." In: Schaffer, H. R. (ed.) *The origins of human social relations* (Academic Press, London 1971) 147-61.
10. Sander, L. W., "Comments on regulations and organisation in the early infant caretaker system." In: Robinson R. J. (ed.) *Brain & Early Behaviour* (Academic Press, London 1969) 311-33.

CHAPTER 4

Simple Sleep Problems

1. Moore, T. & Ucko L., "Night waking in early childhood," *Archives of Disease in Childhood* (1957) 333-342.
2. Laird, D. & Drexel, H., "Experiments with foods and sleep," J. Am. Dietetic Assn. (1934) X: 89-99.
3. Yogman, M. & Zeisel, S., "Diet and sleep patterns in newborn infants," *N. Engl. J. Med* (1983) 309: 1147-9.
4. Illingworth, R. S., *The Normal Child* (Churchill Livingstone, Edinburgh 1979) 28.
5. Paradise, J. L., "Maternal and other factors in the etiology of infantile colic," J. Am. Med. Ass. (1966) 197, 191.
6. Hide, D. W., Guyer, B. M., "Prevalence of Infant Colic," *Archives of Disease in Childhood* (1982) 57: 559-60.

7. Illingworth, R. S., "Evening Colic in Infants," *Lancet* (1959) 1119-20.
8. Grunseit, F., "Evaluation of Efficacy of Dicyclomine Hydrochloride syrup in the treatment of infant colic," *Curr. Med. Res. Opin.* (1977) 5: 258.
9. Moore, T., Ucko, L., *Archives of Disease in Childhood* (1957) 333-42.
10. Radbill, S. X., (1965) *Bull. Hist. Med.* 39, 339.
11. Seward, M. H., *Brit. Dent. J.* 127, 457.

CHAPTER 5

Bedtime Difficulties

1. Bax, M., "Sleep Disturbance in the Young Child," *B.M.J.* (1980) 1177-9.
2. Newson, J. & Newson, E., *Four Years Old in an Urban Community* (Pelican Books, 1970).
3. Southwell, P., Evans, C., Hunt, J., "Effect of a hot milk drink on movements during sleep," *B.M.J.* (1972) 2, 429-31.
4. Fara, J. W. et al, *Science,* 165, 110.
5. Brezinova, V., Oswald, L., "Sleep after a Bedtime Beverage," *B.M.J.* (1972) 2, 432-3.
6. Goldberg, P., Kaufman, D., *Natural Sleep* (Rodale Press, 1978).
7. Ambrose, J. A., *Stimulation in early infancy* (Academic Press, London 1970).
8. Morooka, H., *Sleep gently in the womb* (Toshiba EMI Ltd., Tokyo).
9. Wallechinsky, D. et al, *The Book of Lists* (1980) 2: 232.

CHAPTER 6

Disturbed Nights

1. Newson, J. & Newson, E. *Four Years Old in an Urban Community* (Pelican Books, 1970).

CHAPTER 7

Restless Sleep

1. Anthony, E. J., "An experimental approach to the psychpathology of childhood sleep," *British Journal of Medical Psychology* (1959) 32, 19-37.

2. Anders, T. and Weinstein, P., "Sleep and its Disorders in Infants and Children," *Pediatrics,* (August 1972) Vol. 50, No. 2.
3. Kimmins, C. W., *Children's Dreams* (Longman's Green, London 1920).
4. Illingworth, R. and Illingworth, C., *Babies and Young Children* (Churchill Livingstone 6th Edition), 188.
5. Herbert, M., *Problems of Childhood* (Pan 1975).
6. Bakwin, H., "Sleep Walking in Twins," *Lancet* (1970) Vol. 2: 446-7.
7. Kales, A. et al, "Hereditary Factors in Sleep Walking and Night Terrors," *Brit. Journal of Psychiatry* (1980) 137: 111-8.
8. Bixler, et al, "Prevalence of Sleep Disorders in the Los Angeles Metropolitan Area," *Am. Journal of Psychiatry* 136, 1257-62.
9. "Unquiet Sleep," leading article in *B.M.J.* (1980) 1660-1.

CHAPTER 8

Bed-wetting

1. Newson, John and Elizabeth, *Four Years Old in an Urban Community* (Pelican Books, 1970).
2. Douglas, J. W. B., "Natural History of Enuresis," *B.M.J.* (1976) ii, 233-5.
3. Apley, J., MacKeith, M., *The Child and His Symptoms* (Blackwell Scientific Publications, 1968).
4. Werry, J. C., "Enuresis—a psychosomatic entity?" *Can. Med. Ass. J.* 97, 319.
5. Graham, P. In Kolvin, I., MacKeith, R. C. and Meadow, S. R. (1973), "Bladder Control & Enuresis," *Clinics in Developmental Medicine* (Heinemann) Nos. 48 & 49.
6. Stayte, D. J., "Treatment of Nocturnal Enuresis in a child using hypnosis," *J. Mat. Child Health* (1982) 7: 410-2.
7. Dische, S., *Practitioner* (1978) 221: 323-30.
8. Malem, H., Knapp, M. S., Hiller, E. J., "Electronic Bed-wetting Alarm & Toilet Trainer," *B.M.J.* (1982) 285: 22.
9. *Archives of Disease in Childhood* (1982) 57, 137.

CHAPTER 9

Special Cases—The sleep problems of the handicapped, the hyperactive and the gifted

1. Tucker, I. G., McArthur, K., "The sleep patterns of pre-school hearing impaired children," *J. Br. Assoc. Teachers of the Deaf* (1977) 1: 2-7.

2. Tait, T., Firth, H., "Sleep Problems in Mental Subnormality," *Nursing Mirror* (15th July, 1976).
3. Stare, F. et al, *Pediatrics* 66: 4, 521-5.
4. Hill, P., "The overactive child," *J. Mat. Child Health.* Vol. 4: 86-90.
5. Bidder, R. T. et al, "Behaviour treatment of hyperactive children," *Archives of Disease in Childhood* (1978) 53: 574-9.
6. Bunday, S., "Struggling through the days and nights," *Nursing Mirror* (30th Oct. 1980) iv-v.

CHAPTER 10

Bed-sharing

1. Tine Thevenin, *The Family Bed* (Minneapolis, Minnesota, 1976).
2. Rosemary Ellis, *Motherhood* (Barrie & Jenkins 1977).
3. Zorach, J. Schwartz, A. H. *JAMA* Vol. 244, No. 13: 1498.
4. Crook, W., *JAMA* Vol. 245, No. 4: 343.
5. Kaplan, S., Poznaski, E., "Child Psychiatric Patients who share a bed with a parent," *J Am Acad. Child Psychiatry* (1974) 2: 344-56.
6. Klackenberg, G., "Sleep Behaviour Studied Longitudinally," *Acta Paediatr Scand* (1982) 71: 501-6.

CHAPTER 11

Behavior Therapy

1. Sanger, S., Weir, K., Churchill, E., "Treatment of Sleep Problems: The use of behaviour modification techniques by Health Visitors," *Health Visitor* (1981) 5: 421-4.
2. Richamn, N., "Sleep Problems in Young Children," *Archives of Disease in Childhood* (1981) 56: 491-3.
3. Douglas, J., "Sleep Problems in Children," *Update* (1983) 27: 1239-44.

CHAPTER 12

Sleeping Drugs

1. Ounsted, M. K., Hendrick, A. M., "The first born child: patterns of development," *Devop. Med. Child Neurol.* (1977) 19: 446-53.
2. Illingworth, R. S., *The Normal Child* (Churchill Livingstone, Edinburgh 1979) 254.
3. Valman, H. B., *B.M.J.* (283) 6288: 422-3.
4. Richman, N., "Sleep Problems in Children," *Archives of Disease in Childhood* (1981) 56, 491-3.

5. Powell, B. W., "Sleep Disorders in Childhood," *Practitioner* 208: 198-202.

CHAPTER 13

Who else can help?

1. Chavin, W., Tinson, S., "Children with Sleep Difficulties," *Health Visitor* 53: 477-80.
2. Richards, M., Bernal, J., "Why Some Babies Don't Sleep," *New Society* (28 Feb. 1974).
3. Gibson, H. B., *Hypnosis, its nature and therapeutic uses* (Peter Owen 1977) 176.

INDEX

◆